NATURALLY HEALTHY SKIN

Tips and Techniques for a Lifetime of Radiant Skin

STEPHANIE TOURLES

STOREY BOOKS

Schoolhouse Road
Pownal, Vermont 05261

The mission of Storey Communications is to serve our customers by publishing practical information that encourages personal independence in harmony with the environment.

Edited by Deborah Balmuth and Nancy Ringer
Text design by Susan Bernier (based on an original design
  by Carol Jessop, Black Trout Design)
Text production by Deborah Daly and Erin Lincourt
Cover art & design by Carol Jessop, Black Trout Design
Herb illustrations by Laura Tedeschi
Line drawings by Alison Kolesar
Indexed by Peggy Holloway

Printed in the United States by R.R. Donnelley
10 9 8 7 6 5 4 3 2 1

Library of Congress Cataloging-in-Publication Data

Tourles, Stephanie, 1962–
      Naturally Healthy Skin : tips and techniques for a lifetime of radiant skin / Stephanie Tourles.
            p.   cm.
      ISBN 1-58017-130-3 (pb : alk. paper)
      1. Skin—Care and hygiene. 2. Beauty, Personal. 3. Herbal cosmetics. I. Title.
      RL87.T68 1999
      646.7'26—dc21   99-13151
                                                                                    CIP

DEDICATION

To my grandparents:
Earl and Phenie Ashe
and
Grace and the late Jack Anchors

CONTENTS

FOREWORD

The field of esthetics is growing at a phenomenal rate, and today, care of the skin is more closely linked to the esthetician than ever before. With the aging of the baby boomer generation and the resulting interest in the "medicalization of the beauty industry," the esthetician is being called upon to supply answers to a number of concerns about maintaining healthy skin. In salons, spas, and wellness and medical clinics around the world, estheticians are now performing skin care services that extend well beyond pampering and facials to include total body care as well as more aggressive treatments for scarring and the signs of aging.

Fortunately, the esthetician has always been interested in integrating natural remedies with professional skin care techniques. As consumers become more savvy about skin care products — ingredients, safety, and efficacy — we can expect that the evolution of product development and application will continue to be dictated by the desire for more natural ingredients. On a professional level, we call this struggle and search for information "integrative medicine." For consumers, it means taking their concern for maintaining healthy, translucent skin with natural ingredients into their own hands and homes and becoming increasingly better informed.

With *Naturally Healthy Skin,* Stephanie Tourles offers consumers a very natural approach to beautiful skin. As a graduate of the 600-Hour Advanced Skin Care Program at the Catherine Hinds Institute, she has taken the basic philosophy of the Institute — that healthy skin is directly related to proper skin care, sound nutrition, and a sensible wellness program — to new heights. Her holistic and healthful recipes ensure a lifetime of beautiful skin — naturally!

— AN HINDS, Director of the
Catherine Hinds Institute of Esthetics

ACKNOWLEDGMENTS

My heartfelt appreciation goes out to the following people and organizations for their contributions of knowledge, expertise, wisdom, and technical and emotional support during the writing of this book: my husband, Bill — without our partnership, I would not be who I've become; the invaluable Deborah Balmuth and Nancy Ringer, my editors extraordinaire; Bill and Sylvia Varney for their delicious cookie recipes; Janice Semprini, my beautiful friend, for making me laugh until my stomach hurt; the American Academy of Dermatology; the Skin Cancer Foundation; the American Cancer Society; the National Eczema Association for Science and Education; the National Psoriasis Foundation; the National Rosacea Society; Stephan Brown, for his humor, poetry, and herbal remedies; Melanie Von Zabuesnig, Jean Argus, Julie Bailey, Shatoiya de la Tour, and Debra St. Claire, M.H., for their herbal wisdom and recipes; Melissa Farris, for her invaluable aromatherapy education; Lozetta DeAngelo, fellow esthetician and skin care mentor; Donna Peri, friend and head esthetician, for a fantastic facial and massage — my skin, mind, and body thank you; An Hinds, esthetician and administrator of the Catherine Hinds Institute of Esthetics; Dr. William W. Fiske, M.D., for his advice; and Rosemary Gladstar, for her recipe contribution and United Plant Savers information.

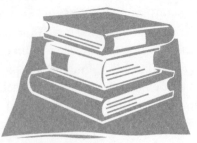

INTRODUCTION

"Smoother, younger-looking skin in seven days. Guaranteed or your money back." How many times have you fallen for that marketing ploy? Most cosmetic companies are very adept at knowing which buttons to push to entice you to purchase their merchandise and empty your wallet, in a flash, with promises of restored youth. The department store counters beckon with their glamorous posters, beautifully made-up salespeople, and buy-one-get-one-free offers. These companies prey on your emotions, all in the guise of making you look and feel better about yourself.

The cosmetics and bodycare industry is made up of many multimillion-dollar corporations. They are in business to make money, and indeed they do. Skin care products have one of the highest price mark-ups of any commodity on the market. Don't get me wrong, though — there are some companies whose products actually do produce the desired results and whose prices are not overly inflated. You will generally find their skin care wares in better health food stores or from a salon or spa that puts a strong emphasis on premium natural ingredients in the products they represent.

It's my belief that an educated consumer is a discerning consumer. In this book, I hope to educate you as to what constitutes a good versus a bad cosmetic. You'll learn about skin form and function, its needs, and how those needs can be met by various herbs, oils, and other natural ingredients. You'll be armed with the knowledge of what to look for in a commercial product as well as how to make your own formulas.

It's only natural to want to look your best, to make a positive, lasting impression upon the people that you greet. When you look good, you feel good. You project an air of confidence. When you are dissatisfied with your appearance, your self-esteem suffers.

Ever had a day when it's an absolute must that you look super for an important event, only to have an unexpected blemish appear in the middle of your forehead or on the tip of your nose, or have a rash develop on your neck? Your skin doesn't always cooperate the way you want it to — especially *when* you want it to. It reacts to emotional upheavals, stress, weather, makeup, dirt, grease, food, and hormones. Remember the Murphy's Law of skin care: If something can flare up, it will . . . and at the most inopportune time!

When your skin looks good, it's translucent, luminous, radiant, and simply exudes glowing health. When it's behaving badly, it's upsetting and occasionally disfiguring, resulting in acne scars, scaly patches, broken capillaries, puffiness, rashes, eczema, or warts. Your potentially beautiful skin can become downright unattractive and ugly from lack of "sun sense." Accumulated sun exposure, over the years, will produce a slew of leathery wrinkles and age spots, which in and of themselves are depressing, but additionally, the incidence of skin cancer is rapidly on the rise. It's not pretty and can be fatal.

Naturally Healthy Skin takes a holistic approach to skin care: Health within is reflected by beautiful skin without. I'll show you how to integrate nutrition, stress reduction, and herbs and other natural ingredients to help systemically remedy your skin care concerns, instead of merely treating the exterior symptoms as is the common approach. Combine this knowledge with a proper cleansing routine and sound sun protection and you'll have the recipe for a lifetime of fabulous looking skin.

Here's to looking and feeling beautiful or handsome, naturally. God Bless!

CHAPTER 1
Up Close and Personal with Your Skin

▼▼▼

As a licensed esthetician (skin-care specialist), I'm fascinated by the workings of the human body, particularly the skin. One of my favorite and most tattered books is *Principles of Anatomy and Physiology,* 4th edition, by Gerard Tortora and Nicholas Anagnostakos. In it they state, "An aggregation of tissues that performs a specific function is an organ. The skin and its derivatives, such as hair, nails, glands, and several specialized receptors, constitute the integumentary system of the body. The skin or cutis is an organ because it consists of tissues structurally joined together to perform specific activities. It is not just a simple thin covering that keeps the body together and gives it protection. The skin is quite complex in structure and performs several functions essential for survival."

Your skin is truly a marvel and an integral part of your being. It is one of the largest organs of the body and definitely the heaviest. Your skin is constantly transmitting and receiving information. If something is amiss, your skin displays signs of interior or exterior distress. If all is well on the homefront, it displays radiance and inner harmony.

STRUCTURE

Your skin — the ultimate wash-and-wear protective barrier — is nothing short of amazing! Just as there are many facets to your personality that, together, form the unique person that you are, there are many layers and structures within your skin that, as a unit, keep this organ running smoothly.

Your skin varies greatly in thickness, with the skin on your eyelids being the thinnest — thinner even than the paper these words are printed on — and the skin on the soles of your feet and your palms the thickest — up to one-fifth of an inch. If you're of average size (125 to 175 pounds) your skin weighs approximately 5 to 8 pounds and if stretched out flat would cover an area of approximately 17 to 20 square feet.

SKINFORMATION

The skin's unbelievable complexity is partially indicated
when we consider the fact that each square inch contains:

- 65 hairs
- 95–100 sebaceous glands
- 78 yards (70 meters) of nerves
- 19 yards (17 meters) of blood vessels
- 650 sweat glands
- 9,500,000 cells
- 1,300 nerve endings (to record pain)
- 19,500 sensory cells at the ends of nerve fibers
- 78 sensory apparatuses for heat
- 13 sensory apparatuses for cold

— Adapted from *Standard Textbook for
Professional Estheticians*, 5th edition, by Joel Gerson

Epidermis

Of the three layers of skin — epidermal, dermal, and subcutaneous — the epidermal layer, or epidermis, is the most visible and thinnest layer and it contains no blood vessels. It's
the part of the skin that wrinkles, breaks out, flakes, and
gets sunburns, blisters, and freckles.

The epidermis consists of five layers:

1. Stratum corneum. The outermost layer consisting
of dead keratinized (toughened or hardened protein) squamous cells that are constantly being shed. This layer forms
a protective shield against bacteria, chemicals, ultraviolet
radiation, heat, and other harmful invaders. It also keeps us
relatively waterproof.

2. Stratum lucidum. A clear layer that reflects light.
This layer is present only in the soles of the feet and palms
of the hands where there are no hair follicles.

3. Stratum granulosum. This layer consists of flat-
tened, almost dead squamous cells that look like tiny granules. These cells contain a dark, staining substance called
keratohyalin, which is involved in keratin formation.

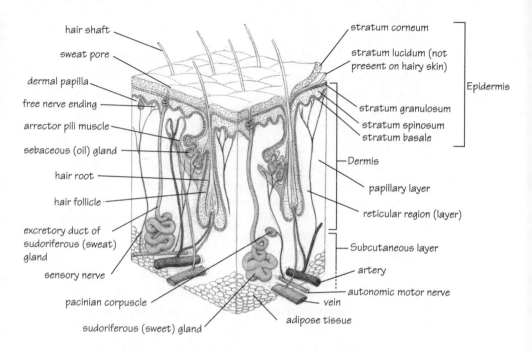

hair shaft

sweat pore

dermal papilla

free nerve ending

arrector pili muscle

sebaceous (oil) gland

hair root

hair follicle

excretory duct of sudoriferous (sweat) gland

sensory nerve

pacinian corpuscle

sudoriferous (sweet) gland

stratum corneum

stratum lucidum (not present on hairy skin)

Epidermis

stratum granulosum

stratum spinosum

stratum basale

Dermis

papillary layer

reticular region (layer)

Subcutaneous layer

artery

autonomic motor nerve

vein

adipose tissue

A cross-section of the skin allows you to see the different layers and how they function.

4. Stratum spinosum. Also called the "prickle layer" because of its spiny appearance under a microscope, the stratum spinosum contains rows of polyhedral (many-sided) cells. Some new skin cell germination takes place here.

5. Stratum basale. This is the basal or base layer that lies next to the dermis. Keratinocytes (keratin-forming cells) and melanocytes (pigment cells) are formed in this layer. As these cells multiply, they gradually push their way up through the above four layers and lose much of their softness and water content. Eventually they dry out, toughen, and die, reaching the stratum corneum where they are sloughed off through a process called desquamation (removal of squamous cells).

SKINFORMATION

Keratin is a protein manufactured by keratinocytes (epidermal cells). Hard keratin makes up hair, feathers, nails, beaks, and horns. Soft keratin makes up epidermal skin.

Dermis

The dermis, also known as the corium or true skin, is a tough, elastic layer of connective tissue. Its abundant blood supply puts roses in your cheeks and gives you a look of vitality. This strong second layer basically holds everything together.

The dermis consists of two layers:

1. Papillary. Lying beneath the epidermis, it binds the epidermis and dermis together. This layer comprises about one-fifth of the total thickness of the dermis. It contains small, fingerlike, highly vascular projections called "papillae" (better known as the ridges that comprise your fingerprints and footprints), which point upward into the epidermis. These projections contain capillaries and nerve endings that are supersensitive to touch stimuli. This layer contains connective tissue and elastic fibers closely bound together.

2. Reticular. The reticular layer houses bundles of interlaced collagenous fibers interspersed with coarse elastic fibers. These meshlike fibers give the skin its strength, elasticity, and ability to stretch and bounce back to its original shape. As we age, it is this quality that gradually diminishes. Our skin loses its spring or tone and begins to wrinkle, sag, and stiffen. Collagen formation slows as we enter our thirties. This layer also contains fat cells, blood and lymph vessels, oil and sweat glands, arrector pili muscles (these give you goose bumps), and hair follicles.

Subcutaneous Tissue

Subcutaneous means "beneath the skin." This is the fatty layer that lies beneath the dermis and connects to the underlying muscle tissue. A little fat is a good thing, as far as your skin is concerned. It acts as a shock absorber and insulator protecting your internal organs and gives your skin a smooth, strong foundation. Too much fat is not a good thing, but a little bit keeps your face from looking drawn and hollow and gives it beautiful contours. This layer becomes thinner as we age (or crash diet), leaving behind sagging, unsupported skin.

FUNCTION

Our skin performs many vital functions on which our lives depend:

- Helps the body maintain a steady temperature
- Protects us from physical, chemical, biological, thermal, and electrical damage
- Prevents excessive loss of minerals
- Acts as a moisture regulator, preventing excessive entry and evaporation of water
- Serves as a highly sensitive sensory organ, responding to heat, cold, pain, pleasure, and pressure
- Assists in processes of excretion via sweating, eliminating salts, urea, water, and other toxins
- Secretes sebum (oil secreted by the sebaceous glands), which lubricates the skin and keeps it from drying out
- Metabolizes and stores fat
- Converts ultraviolet rays into vitamin D, which helps maintain strong bones by enhancing calcium absorption

As a general rule, your skin is designed to keep more things out than it lets in. Certain substances, including antibiotics, essential oils, vitamins, fat-soluble hormones, and fatty substances such as creams and oils, can be absorbed through the pores and hair follicles. Infection-causing bacteria usually enter the skin through cuts, pimples, boils, and acne.

In addition to its regulatory functions, the skin also has the responsibility of showcasing a certain aesthetic appeal. In a society that often passes judgment based on "first appearances," we cannot overlook the appealing aspect of a healthy, vibrant complexion. More often than not, our look is the basis for social acceptance. The condition of our skin, the most noticeable and visible of organs, affects our self-confidence and, in turn, how our presence is perceived by others. Billions of dollars are spent each year to improve the skin's appearance even though basic, natural care is all that's really necessary to keep this complex organ running at peak performance.

CHAPTER 2
Super Foods and Other Essentials for a Fabulous Face and Body

Nutrition is so very important with skin care. What you eat is reflected on your face. In my daily quest for natural beauty, health, and vitality, I'm always in awe of what Mother Nature has to offer. She provides everything you need to encourage and support the healthy functioning of your skin, but it's up to you to partake of these offerings. I recommend that you try to eat a balanced diet of minimally processed whole foods in their natural state. Include approximately 40–60 percent complex carbohydrates, 20–30 percent lean protein, and 10–20 percent fat, depending upon your activity level and state of wellness.

On the following pages you'll learn how to nourish the very foundation of your skin and improve your well-being.

ESSENTIAL VITAMINS

Powerhouse vitamins — that's what I call the vitamins outlined below. They provide a potent combination of antioxidants and healing agents that boost your skin's ability to make you look your glowing best.

VITAMIN A (BETA-CAROTENE)
Description: Fat-soluble antioxidant
Outstanding Sources: Liver (fish liver oil, especially), blue-green algae, pumpkin and winter squashes, alfalfa, carrots, cayenne pepper, dandelion greens, parsley, spinach, apricots, beet greens, broccoli, sweet potatoes, kale, lettuce, endive, cantaloupe, watermelon, tomatoes
Skin Care Benefits: Essential for growth and maintenance of epithelial (skin) tissue and proper functioning of mucous membranes. Helps prevent dry, rough skin and premature

aging. Speeds healing, especially of acne, impetigo, vision problems. Boosts immunity.

Deficiency Symptoms: Premature wrinkles; acne; pimples; blackheads; psoriasis; vision disorders; respiratory problems; dry, rough, thick, itchy, scaly, cracked skin; slowed healing. An early symptom of deficiency is "chicken skin" — small raised bumps on the back of the neck, upper arms, back, and shoulders.

B-COMPLEX VITAMINS

Description: Water-soluble nutrients. The B vitamins — thiamine, riboflavin, niacin, B_6, B_{12}, folate, pantothenate, PABA, inositol, biotin, and choline — are grouped together as a complex because when naturally occurring, they are always found together — you would never find one of the B vitamins isolated in a substance. If you must supplement, be sure to take one that supplies the entire complex.

Outstanding Sources: Lean beef, chicken, egg yolks, liver, milk, brewer's yeast, whole grains, alfalfa, almonds, sunflower seeds, soy products, green leafy vegetables, blue-green algae, fresh wheat germ, molasses, peas, beans

Skin Care Benefits: The antistress vitamin! Helps prevent premature aging and acne. Promotes healthy circulation and metabolism. Essential for wound healing (sunburn, bruises, infections). Aids new cell growth. Increases vitality.

Deficiency Symptoms: Sore mouth and lips, eczema, skin lesions, dandruff, pale complexion, pigmentation problems, premature wrinkles

VITAMIN C

Description: Water-soluble antioxidant

Outstanding Sources: Rose hips, citrus fruits, tomatoes, berries, pineapple, apples, persimmons, acerola cherries, broccoli, green leafy vegetables, potatoes, bell and hot peppers, currants, papayas

Skin Care Benefits: Helps produce collagen in connective tissue. Strengthens capillary walls, speeds healing, and helps battle environmental stress and toxins.

Deficiency Symptoms: Bruises, spongy gums, wrinkles, sagging skin, premature aging, pyorrhea, slowed healing

VITAMIN D

Description: Fat soluble nutrient

Outstanding Sources: Fish liver oils, herring, mackerel, salmon, tuna, fortified milk, fortified soy milk, alfalfa, watercress, egg yolks, sunshine

Skin Care Benefits: Combined with vitamin A, helps treat acne. Treats herpes simplex, slows premature aging, enhances bone mineralization and calcium absorption.

Deficiency Symptoms: Lack of vitality, slow growth, osteomalacia, osteoporosis, rickets

VITAMIN E

Description: Fat-soluble antioxidant

Outstanding Sources: Cold-pressed vegetable oils, whole grains, eggs, alfalfa, parsley, sprouted seeds and nuts, fresh wheat germ, green leafy vegetables

Skin Care Benefits: Oxygenates tissues, increases body's stores of vitamin A, protects tissues of skin and eyes, slows premature aging, blocks formation of tumors, speeds healing of severe burns and chronic skin lesions. May decrease scarring. Promotes red blood cell formation, and may be beneficial in cases of lupus.

Deficiency Symptoms: Degeneration of epithelial cells in the organs and skin-germinating cells (resulting in tissue membrane instability and collagen shrinkage), premature aging, lackluster skin, lethargy, increased tendency to bruise as a result of the fragility of red blood cells

ESSENTIAL MINERALS

Minerals are the building blocks of gorgeous skin. Four minerals in particular are necessary for the proper growth of healthy, luminous, resilient skin: iodine, silicon, sulfur, and zinc.

IODINE

Outstanding Sources: Fish, shellfish, blue-green algae, sunflower seeds, kelp, iodized salt, sea salt

Skin Care Benefits: Aids in healing skin infections, increases oxygen consumption and metabolic rate in the skin. Helps prevent roughness and premature wrinkling.

Deficiency Symptoms: Slowed growth and healing, slowed metabolism, poor skin tone, dry skin
Contraindication: Iodine may aggravate acneic skin.

SILICON

Outstanding Sources: Horsetail, blue-green algae, nettle, echinacea root, dandelion root, alfalfa, kelp, flaxseed, oat straw, barley grass, wheat grass, apples, berries, burdock root, beets, onions, almonds, peanuts, sunflower seeds, grapes
Skin Care Benefits: Aids in collagen formation, keeps skin taut, strengthens bones and skin tissues, helps prevent wrinkles.
Deficiency Symptoms: Premature wrinkles, lack of skin tone, sagging skin

SULFUR

Outstanding Sources: Turnips, dandelion greens, radishes, horseradish, string beans, onions, garlic, cabbage, celery, kale, watercress, soybeans, fresh fish, lean meats, eggs, asparagus
Skin Care Benefits: Called "the beauty mineral." Helps keep skin clear and smooth.
Deficiency Symptoms: Dry scalp, rashes, eczema, acne

ZINC

Outstanding Sources: Blue-green algae, barley grass, alfalfa, yellow dock root, echinacea root, kelp, dulse, fresh wheat germ, pumpkin seeds, sunflower seeds, brewer's yeast, milk, eggs, fish, oysters, green leafy vegetables, onions, beans, nuts
Skin Care Benefits: Aids in wound healing, promotes cell growth, boosts immunity, and helps treat acne when combined with vitamins A and B.
Deficiency Symptoms: Slow healing, dandruff, lowered resistance to infections

ESSENTIAL FATS AND FATTY ACIDS

Fat in the diet is vital to your skin's health and beauty. Without fat, your skin has no contour, no roundness. It can't be beautiful without at least a thin layer of padding to support it and give it shape. Fat is a necessary requirement if radiant, moisturized skin is what you seek.

Fat is comprised mainly of substances called fatty acids. There are three types of fatty acids: saturated, monounsaturated, and polyunsaturated.

Saturated fatty acids are easy to recognize because they are solid at room temperature. They occur in foods such as butter; coconut and palm oils; beef, chicken, and pork fat; and full-fat dairy products. Saturated fat is manufactured by your body, but the excess that you consume can lead to an increased risk of high cholesterol and heart disease.

Monounsaturated fatty acids are liquid at room temperature and found in such foods as olive oil, canola oil, cashews, avocados, and oily cold-water fish such as bluefish, swordfish, halibut, mackerel, and salmon. These fatty acids may actually be beneficial for your heart in that they do not elevate your cholesterol and may help reduce it.

Polyunsaturated fatty acids are similar to monounsaturated fatty acids and are also liquid at room temperature, but have a slightly different molecular structure. Polyunsaturated fatty acids are found predominantly in foods such as flax seeds, walnuts, and oily cold-water fish, as well as safflower, sunflower, and corn oils. However, high amounts of these oils, especially the less expensive, highly refined brands sold in many grocery stores, have been associated with an increased risk of certain types of cancer. If you're frying or cooking, I'd recommend olive or canola oil over the oils high in polyunsaturated fatty acids

Monounsaturated fatty acids and polyunsaturated fatty acids, in particular, contain essential fatty acids (EFAs). Cliff Sheats, author of *Lean Bodies,* writes, "All EFAs are vitamin-like substances that have a protective effect on the body. The reason these fats are called 'essential' is because your body cannot manufacture them; you must obtain them from the foods you eat. EFAs are the 'good guys' in the nutrition story."

Only a very small amount of fat is needed to meet basic nutritional needs. As little as 2 to 3 teaspoons (10–15 ml) a day of polyunsaturated fat will provide all the EFA's your body needs.

As far as skin care goes, there are two types of EFAs that are greatly beneficial.

OMEGA-3

Outstanding Sources: Cold-water fish such as bluefish, salmon, mackerel, and tuna; ground flax seeds; flaxseed oil (sometimes called the "vegetable alternative to fish oil"); walnuts and walnut oil; Brazil nuts

Skin Care Benefits: Proper wound healing, reported to relieve arthritis symptoms, soften and aid in healing eczema and psoriasis, balances sebum production.

Deficiency Symptoms: Dry, scaly skin; eczema; inflammatory skin conditions; slow healing

OMEGA-6

Constituent: Gamma-linolenic acid (GLA)

Outstanding Sources: Evening primrose oil, borage oil, black currant oil, blue-green algae

Skin Care Benefits: Promotes smooth, healthy, moisturized skin and proper joint function and flexibility.

Deficiency Symptoms: Dry and flaky skin, eczema, painful joints, stiffness

WHOLE FOOD SUPPLEMENTS

Ever visit a lovely, tranquil farm and see the beautiful vitamin-pill trees growing in the orchard down by the brook? Of course not! We're so busy these days that we've become a nation of pill poppers. We swallow our "one-a-day" in an effort to ensure that we get a nutritious and balanced diet. We consume so much fast food and junk food that many of us seem to think that a fractionated, synthetically derived pill will fill the gaps in our diets. Not so!

Sure, laboratory-made vitamin and mineral supplements have their rightful place in certain disease conditions and deficiencies, but for general health and well-being, consumption of whole, unprocessed foods as Mother Nature presents them is the way to go. Additionally, naturally derived supplements such as herbal capsules, tinctures, teas, syrups, brewer's yeast, and blue-green algae, to name a few, are wonderful, nutrient-dense foods to include in your beautiful-skin regimen.

The recipes that follow are chock-full of easily absorbable vitamins and minerals. They'll also provide you with a delicious way to boost your energy levels as well as your natural immunity.

SKIN-SATIONAL HERB TEA

A tasty blend for an infusion that, hot or cold, helps replenish a deficient system and restore lackluster skin. All herbs in this formula are in dried form.

2 tablespoons (30 ml) lemon balm
1 tablespoon (15 ml) lavender flowers
1 tablespoon (15 ml) peppermint
1 tablespoon (15 ml) chamomile flowers
1 tablespoon (15 ml) rose petals
1 tablespoon (15 ml) nettle
1 tablespoon (15 ml) alfalfa
1 tablespoon (15 ml) rose hips
2 teaspoons (10 ml) dandelion leaves
2 teaspoons (10 ml) raspberry leaves
½ teaspoon (2½ ml) gingerroot

To make: Combine all herbs in a medium-size bowl and stir to blend. Store in a tightly sealed tin, jar, or plastic tub or bag away from light in a cool, dry location. Best if used within 6 months.
To use: Bring a cup of water to a boil in a small saucepan. Remove from heat and add 1 teaspoon (5 ml) of tea. Cover and allow to steep for 10–15 minutes. Strain before drinking. Add honey, cream, or lemon if desired.
Yield: Approximately 30 cups
(7½ liters) of tea

Skin-So-Smoothie

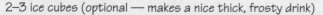

I refer to this recipe as my "antistress breakfast boost" formula. It's loaded with complexion-enhancing, stress-reducing B vitamins, calcium, potassium, zinc, iron, fiber, protein, and complex carbohydrates for sustained energy. I love the taste, but if you're not crazy about about brewer's yeast, the flavor will take a bit of getting used to.

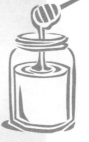

   1 frozen banana or 1 cup (250 ml) frozen strawberries
   2 cups (500 ml) low-fat milk or fortified soy milk
   1 tablespoon (15 ml) brewer's yeast
   2 teaspoons (10 ml) blackstrap molasses
   2 teaspoons (10 ml) raw sunflower seeds
   1 teaspoon (5 ml) raw sesame seeds
  10 raw almonds
   ¼ cup (60 ml) raw or cooked oatmeal
   2 teaspoons (10 ml) honey
   ¼ teaspoon (4 ml) ground cinnamon
 2–3 ice cubes (optional — makes a nice thick, frosty drink)

To make: Combine all ingredients in blender and whiz on high until smooth for about 30–60 seconds total.
To use: I usually consume the entire batch throughout the morning hours, taking sips between my work projects. Alternatively, pour half the recipe into a mug, cover, and refrigerate the rest until later in the day.
Yield: Makes approximately two 1½-cup (375 ml) servings or 1 large meal

These next two recipes were graciously donated by Bill and Sylvia Varney, owners of the Fredericksburg Herb Farm in Fredericksburg, Texas (see resources). This herb farm, spa, and restaurant is simply beautiful — an oasis under the hot Texas sun!

The Varneys say, "For healthy hair and skin, what goes *in* the body comes before what goes *on* it. The skin, like every other part of the body, receives its nourishment from the bloodstream. Overload your body with caffeine, alcohol, cigarettes, refined sugar, saturated fat, emotional stress, and guess what? Poor color, circles under the eyes, blemished skin, and a never-ending bad hair day. Take a nibble, boost your body and your spirits with a cookie.

"Surprised?" ask the Varneys, "Our cookie recipes are different! They are dense in nutrients, without the abundance of fat and refined sweeteners found in ordinary cookies. They're rich in B vitamins to nourish your nerves and put a sparkle in your eyes; rich in calcium to strengthen your bones; rich in iron for your blood; rich in fiber to clean out your insides; and rich in potassium for your heart too. Best of all, you'll find that in the pursuit of health, vigor, and beauty, your taste buds never had it so good!"

SKINFORMATION

"Skin must be nourished from the inside. The skin receives its nutrition through the bloodstream from nutrients absorbed through the gastrointestinal tract. Actually, the skin receives up to one-third of the blood circulating in the body," states D'Lynne Miller, owner of the Eden Spa in McLean, Virginia, and author of "New Year's Revolution: Reviewing the Fundamentals to Help Clients Fulfill Their Resolutions," published in *Les Nouvelles Esthetiques*, January 1998.

Honey Pecan Cookies

Full of good B vitamins that help you keep your cool, these verbena-scented cookies perk up those afternoon slumps. Nibble one and resist empty-calorie temptations.

1 cup (250 ml) whole wheat flour
½ cup plus 2 tablespoons (155 ml) unbleached flour
2 tablespoons (30 ml) wheat germ
2 tablespoons (30 ml) bran
2 tablespoons (30 ml) powdered milk
½ teaspoon (2½ ml) baking soda
¼ cup (60 ml) unsalted butter
½ cup (125 ml) honey
1 egg
1 4" (10 cm) sprig lemon verbena, minced, or ½ teaspoon
    (3 ml) dried (or 2 teaspoons [10 ml] minced fresh lemon
    balm leaves, or 2 teaspoons [10 ml] grated lemon zest)
2 tablespoons (30 ml) fresh lemon juice
½ cup (125 ml) buttermilk
½ cup (125 ml) pecans, toasted and finely chopped
Toasted, chopped pecans for garnish

To make:
1. Preheat oven to 325°F (162°C).
2. Stir together all dry ingredients in a bowl.
3. In food processor, beat the butter and honey together, then add egg, lemon verbena, lemon juice, and buttermilk and process until smooth and creamy. Add dry ingredients and mix briefly until incorporated. Pulse in chopped pecans.
4. Drop batter by heaping spoonfuls about 2 inches (5 cm) apart onto an ungreased cookie sheet. Garnish with pecans. Bake for 15–18 minutes. Check cookies frequently, they do burn easily. Remove to wire rack to cool.
To use: Enjoy one for a sweet breakfast or anytime for a quick, energizing, skin-healthy snack.
Yield: Approximately 1 dozen, 200 calories each

Apricot Chews

Each day, eat something that, if planted, would grow — such as the seeds in these no-bake cookies. Apricots and raisins add iron, necessary for the hemoglobin that transports oxygen to cells, giving you a healthy glow. Lecithin granules, available in most health food stores, sharpen the mind and improve memory. Rosemary adds a peppy finish.

12 dried unsulfured apricots, chopped
½ cup (125 ml) raisins
1 cup (250 ml) apple juice
1 4" (10 cm) sprig of rosemary, minced, or ½ teaspoon (3 ml) dried
3 tablespoons (45 ml) almonds, raw or lightly toasted
3 tablespoons (45 ml) low-fat granola cereal
3 tablespoons (45 ml) lecithin granules
3 tablespoons (45 ml) raw or toasted wheat germ
2 tablespoons (30 ml) bran cereal
1 tablespoon (15 ml) dry milk powder
2 tablespoons (30 ml) unsweetened shredded coconut, raw or toasted
2 tablespoons (30 ml) sunflower kernels, raw or toasted
3 tablespoons (45 ml) sesame seeds, raw or toasted
Raw or toasted walnut halves for garnish

To make:
1. In a small saucepan, pour apple juice over apricots and raisins. Simmer uncovered for 30 minutes. Drain.
2. In a food processor, puree the fruit and rosemary.
3. In a separate bowl, blend puree with almonds, granola, lecithin, wheat germ, bran, milk powder, coconut, sunflower kernels, and sesame seeds.
4. Place mixture on waxed or parchment paper or aluminum foil. Using sides of paper, form mixture into a 10–12" (25–30 cm) log. Wrap and refrigerate for an hour. Slice log into 12 pieces. Press a walnut in the center of each slice.
To use: Wrap individually with plastic food wrap and refrigerate to keep firm. Enjoy!
Yield: 1 dozen, approximately 80 calories each.

SWEET 'N' NUTTY SNACK MIX

*C*onvenient and portable. One hundred percent better for you than a candy bar or chips! I often keep a baggie of this mixture in my purse so I don't feel tempted to visit the nearest drive-through window when the munchies hit. This dried fruit and nut trail mix contains the essential fats, proteins, and complex carbohydrates your body craves just before that midafternoon slump kicks in and all the nutrients your skin demands to stay in tip-top shape.

½ cup (125 ml) raw almonds
½ cup (125 ml) raw hazelnuts
½ cup (125 ml) dried, unsulfured, pitted cherries
½ cup (125 ml) large unsulfured raisins
½ cup (125 ml) raw Brazil nuts
¼ cup (60 ml) lightly salted sunflower seeds, toasted
¼ cup (60 ml) lightly salted pumpkin seeds, toasted
¼ cup (60 ml) dried unsulfured apricots, chopped
Dash of cinnamon or nutmeg (optional)

To make: Place all ingredients into a plastic bag or food storage container and shake well. Keep tightly sealed in the refrigerator unless consumed within 2 weeks as raw nuts become rancid quicker than the roasted ones.
To use: Consume a handful or so whenever the snacking mood strikes.
Yield: Approximately 3¼ cups of snack mix.

To Toast or Not to Toast

Toasting nuts, seeds, and coconut does enhance the flavor of these cookies, but also slightly diminishes their nutritional content. If you decide to toast, here's how:

Preheat the oven to 350°F (180°C). Place the ingredients in an ungreased baking pan and bake for 12 to 15 minutes, stirring occasionally, until the contents of the pan begin to turn golden brown. Your kitchen should smell yummy!

FIVE DAILY RITUALS
FOR BEAUTIFUL SKIN

Skin care shouldn't be a complex chore. It should be simple, natural, and basic. And if a few of these straightforward skin care rituals are free for the asking, then so much the better!

I've outlined five of my favorite treatments below. You may be surprised to discover how fundamental these are to achieving glowing skin.

Cleansing Routine

A beauty must! Cleanse your skin twice daily (only once if your skin is dry) using a mild, natural, inexpensive cleanser designed for your skin type. (See chapter 3 for a more in-depth discussion on this topic.)

Cleaning your skin is especially important before going to bed because your body excretes toxins through your skin as you sleep. If facial pores are clogged with makeup and dirt, breakouts can occur. If you perspire a lot in your line of work or you exercise heavily, then rinse off and massage your body with a coarse cloth or loofah before retiring to remove salt and dead skin buildup. Your skin needs to breathe while you sleep!

SKINFORMATION

Sweat is actually good for the skin. It's almost 99 percent water and contains urea and lactic acid, two terrific natural moisturizers that are common ingredients in most moisturizing creams. So go ahead and let 'em see you sweat, it will do your skin a world of good!

Exercise

Try to exercise outside if possible to help oxygenate your cells with fresh air and facilitate waste removal through your skin. If you live in a city, try to find a green space — a park or a greenway — to exercise in. If city streets, with their attendant pollution, is your only outdoor option, exercising in a gym may be a better alternative. Exercises such as walking, biking, rollerblading, and weight lifting improve cardiovascular fitness and muscular endurance, which translates into increased energy and a rosy complexion.

Sleep, Blissful Sleep

Has your "get-up-and-go" got up and gone? Sleep deprivation takes its toll on your face in a hurry. To look and feel your absolute best, you need to get deeply restful, quality sleep. I don't care what else you do to your skin, if you are sleep deprived, your skin will look sallow, dull, tired, and saggy, and with your poor, puffy eyes you will resemble a frog prince or princess. And, of course, your energy level will be less than desirable. Sleep — it's the best-kept skin care secret there is!

Sunlight

Ten to fifteen minutes of daily unprotected exposure to sunlight is essential to the health of your bones and your skin. It helps your body absorb calcium due to the skin's ability to convert the sun's rays into vitamin D. Sun exposure helps heal eczema, psoriasis, and acne, and energizes your body. Its warm rays just make you feel good all over.

Always wear a sunscreen with a high SPF if you are going to be exposed for more than fifteen minutes at a time, especially between the hours of 10:30 A.M. and 4:30 P.M. when the sun's rays are at their strongest.

If your dermatologist advises that you avoid the sun entirely, other sources of vitamin D include egg yolks, fish liver oil, vitamin D–supplemented milk or soy milk, organ meats, salmon, sardines, and herring.

Water

What goes in must go out. Water helps move everything right along. Eight to twelve 8-ounce glasses of pure water a day combined with a fibrous diet will help cleanse your body of toxins and keep your colon functioning as it should. Impurities not disposed of in a timely manner via the internal organs of elimination (such as the kidneys, liver, lungs, and large intestine), will find an alternate exit, namely your skin, which is sometimes referred to as the "third kidney." Pimples and rashes may develop as your body tries to unload its wastes through your skin. Water also keeps your skin hydrated and moisturized, so drink up!

CHAPTER 3
Skin Care Basics

▼▼▼

Caring for your skin doesn't have to be a complicated affair. It's quite simple, actually — just don't tell the salespeople behind the department store cosmetics counter I said that. Their livelihood depends on the number of bottles of skin-pampering potions you purchase. If they had their way, you'd be buying an eye cream, a lip exfoliating cream, a lip gloss, a lipstick sealer, a throat cream, a diuretic for the puffiness under your eyes, under-eye circle concealer, antiwrinkle cream, skin-lightening lotion, body sloughing cream, bust-enhancing cream, thigh cream, a blackhead/pore-tightening mask, youth serum (once they get it figured out), pre-cleanser, regular cleanser, clarifying lotion, hyperpigmentation spot treatment cream — the list is endless.

Cosmetic companies want to sell you hope in a jar, the hope of fresh, new, wrinkle-free skin and restored youth. Let's face it — it's never going to happen! However, your quest for a vibrant, healthy appearance needn't be terribly expensive or complicated or include a bevy of synthetic chemicals. In this chapter, I'll show you how to identify your skin type and discuss what products are most beneficial. You'll learn how to get down to the basics of simple but effective natural skin care.

KEEP IT SIMPLE

Chapter 2 detailed how nutrition, exercise, sunlight, water consumption, and sleep are vital to a healthy body and clear skin. These factors affect us internally and result in vibrant and glowing skin fortified from the inside out. Your skin must be properly cared for externally as well, but this doesn't mean you have to spend hundreds of dollars every year on the latest synthetic technological skin care breakthrough, or even sixty dollars on a tiny jar of throat firming cream with encapsulated liposomes that burst upon your skin at scheduled intervals.

I believe in a basic skin care routine. Five products — a cleanser, a toner or astringent, a moisturizer, an exfoliant or antioxidant, and a sunscreen — are all anyone, man or woman, needs to use to maintain healthy skin. Find a moisturizing sunscreen, and the number drops to four. Doesn't get much simpler than that!

- ◆ **Cleanser** — to wash away dirt, makeup, toxins, and pollutants
- ◆ **Toner or astringent** — to remove any residual cleanser or oil from the skin and to temporarily refine the appearance of large pores
- ◆ **Moisturizer** — to replenish and minimize wear and tear
- ◆ **Exfoliator or antioxidant** — to refresh and smooth the complexion, such as a gentle facial scrub, alpha- or beta-hydroxy gel or cream, or topical vitamin C
- ◆ **Sunscreen** — to protect

TOP 4 CLEANSING TIPS

1. If you wear foundation, powder, or waterproof face and eye makeup, be sure to cleanse your skin twice. The first cleansing removes the makeup, and the second cleansing removes excess sebum, and dead skin, and deep cleans your pores.

2. Rinse, rinse, rinse. You can never rinse your face and body too much! Cleansing products, massage oil, makeup, and soap can leave a film on your skin that will clog pores.

3. No matter how oily your complexion, limit your cleansing routine to twice a day, to avoid stripping your skin's protective acid mantle.

4. Avoid hot water! Hot water dehydrates and irritates most skin types. Use tepid or warm water only.

DISCOVERING YOUR SKIN TYPE

Granted, maintaining a healthy lifestyle is key to having beautiful skin, but the real secret to having skin that is irresistible to touch and behold is to accurately know your skin type and care for it accordingly. Too many people treat their skin with the wrong products; instead of improving the condition of their skin, they actually worsen it.

To help you identify and evaluate your skin type and understand its special needs, seven different classifications are detailed below. Nine times out of ten you will fall into one of these categories, but some of you may overlap into another category or two. That's okay. Everybody's unique.

Oily Skin

Characteristics: Medium-to-large pores in T-zone area and perhaps on the cheeks, shoulders, neck, chest, and back as well. Overactive sebaceous glands give the skin a slick, shiny appearance within an hour after cleansing. May or may not be prone to acne or pimples, but pores do become clogged easily. Oily skin is not prone to fine lines and wrinkles because it is well-lubricated.

Seasonal Variations: Heat and humidity tend to increase the amount of sebum production whereas cooler temperatures and lower humidity are a boon for oily complexions. Surface dehydration (lack of moisture) may occur in very cold, dry weather.

Cleansing: Use a water-based gel, milk, or clay cleanser that does not dry out the skin's surface twice a day. You may use a gentle, herbal glycerin or goat milk soap if you wish, as long as it does not dry out your skin. Your goal here is to remove the excess oil, but not strip your skin of its protective barrier. "Squeaky clean" is not what you're after!

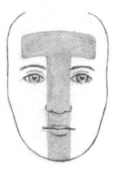

The area of the face that encompasses the forehead, nose, and chin is known as the T-zone.

Overdrying the sur-
face of an oily com-
plexion, it is believed,
may stimulate the
sebaceous glands to
produce more oil —
exactly the opposite
of what you are
trying to achieve!

(If your skin is extremely oily, you may need to bathe your body twice a day, using your preferred cleanser.)

Toning: A gentle, astringent herbal tea such as yarrow, sage, or peppermint will remove any leftover cleanser and dirt from the facial skin. Avoid using isopropyl (rubbing) alcohol; it's too harsh and extremely drying. If you tend to break out or have excessively oily skin on your shoulders, neck, chest, or back, you may want to apply an herbal astringent tea to those areas as often as necessary to remove the oil and freshen your skin.

Moisturizing: Depending on the degree of oiliness, you may not need a moisturizer at all or at the very least, use a light moisturizing aloe vera–based spray or aromatic hydrosol to keep the facial skin's surface hydrated. Apply a light moisturizing lotion to your body if you feel it's needed.

Special Treatments: Use of a clay mask or exfoliating scrub twice a week will discourage formation of blackheads, minimize breakouts, and reduce the appearance of enlarged pores. Alpha- or beta-hydroxy acid treatments, used twice a week, are good to smooth and refine the skin's surface (these products can also be used on oily areas of the body). An herbal facial steam using yarrow, sage, or rosemary with a couple of drops of tea tree essential oil is perfect for disinfecting any minor pimples or open blemishes you may have. For pimples, I recommend an overnight spot treatment mask using 2 to 3 drops of tea tree or thyme (chemotype linalol) essential oil combined with a bit of clay and water to help heal those pesky blemishes. *Note:* Do not use a facial scrub if you have acne, as this can further aggravate the condition.

Normal Skin

Characteristics: Neither too dry nor too oily. Usually free of blemishes, but may form blackheads. May get a little oily in T-zone 4 to 6 hours after cleansing depending on humidity and temperature. Pores are normal in size.

Seasonal Variations: The face tends to be oilier in summer than winter and the entire body may suffer from surface dehydration in very cold weather.

Cleansing: For the face, use a gentle water- or milk-based cleanser that will remove surface impurities without stripping skin of oil twice a day. You can use the same cleanser for your body or a mild natural soap.

Toning: Lavender, rose, rosemary, German chamomile, or orange floral waters refresh and further cleanse the skin.

Moisturizing: A light but protective lotion designed to seal in moisture is recommended for both the face and the body. Avoid anything too heavy as it will cause oiliness.

Special Treatments: For the face, a pore-refining clay mask once a week or a moisturizing mask in winter can be used if necessary. Alpha- or beta-hydroxy acid treatments are recommended twice a week to minimize fine lines and smooth the skin. An herbal facial steam once a week will help cleanse pores.

Dry Skin

Characteristics: Lacks natural oil and moisture, the basic requirements for that healthy glow! May appear flaky or scaly and be rough textured if very dry. Has small pores and feels taut after cleansing. Develops lines and wrinkles more rapidly than any other skin type. Ages prematurely.

Seasonal Variations: Dry skin loves warm temperatures and humidity, but the winter can be a challenge. Cold temperatures and dry air rob the skin of moisture resulting in chapping, irritation, and redness.

Cleansing: For the face, use a moisture-rich cleansing milk or cream twice a day. Avoid soap at all costs. Products enriched with chamomile, calendula, or lavender are nurturing and gentle for this skin type. For your body, I recommend cleansing with a small drawstring bath bag filled with oatmeal. Once wet, the oatmeal will cover your skin with moisturizing "oat milk," which is quite soothing for dry skin.

Toning: The classic rosewater and glycerin lotion makes a perfect toner to help rehydrate and further cleanse thirsty facial skin.

Moisturizing: It is important to use a rich, rapidly absorbing cream or lotion for both the face and the body that will provide a barrier against the harsh, drying environment and keep moisture in the skin where it belongs.

Special Treatments: A fennel seed facial steam once a week will help hydrate the skin and cleanse the pores. Use a moisturizing mask once or twice a week as needed. For both the face and the body, alpha- or beta-hydroxy acid treatments (depending upon your skin's sensitivity) are recommended once a week, as tolerated, to remove dead skin cell build up and promote moisturizer absorption. The nightly use of an emollient eye cream will moisturize the delicate tissue in this area.

Combination Skin

Characteristics: Combination skin results when two skin types occur on one face; there are both dry and oily areas. Generally, the T-zone will appear oily with enlarged pores, visible blackheads, and may be prone to minor breakouts or acne, while the cheeks and neck may feel dry and tight, with possible surface flakiness. Combination skin can be tricky to treat. Most people think that caring for this skin type requires a dual approach, such as using astringent products for the oily areas and moisturizing products for the dry areas. I prefer to use products that regulate and normalize the sebum production for the entire face and throat.

Seasonal Variations: The oily areas tend to normalize a bit in winter while the dry areas get drier. Can be quite aggravating.

Cleansing: A water- or milk-based cleanser used twice a day deep cleans and refines the pores while hydrating and protecting against dryness. Gentle, soap-free products are recommended, especially those containing rosemary, chemotype verbenon, niaouli, everlasting, German chamomile, or spike lavender essential oils.

Toning: To remove excess cleanser, hydrate the skin, and normalize pH, I recommend German chamomile, rose, orange, or lavender floral waters. Four parts yarrow tea mixed with one part vegetable glycerin works wonderfully, too.

Moisturizing: Apply a very light moisturizer all over and apply a bit of nourishing cream to the drier areas if necessary.

Special Treatments: The pores of a combination skin tend to clog easily, thus the dead skin and debris need to be exfoliated on a regular basis. A gentle, pore-refining clay or oatmeal mask followed by an alpha- or beta-hydroxy acid treatment (depending upon your skin's sensitivity) twice a week will be quite beneficial. Once a week, enjoy a lavender and rosemary facial steam to remove impurities from the pores.

Mature Skin

Characteristics: Mature skin usually develops a crepey texture that appears loose and sagging with fine lines and wrinkles. It tends to be dry, but can be normal or oily, and may or may not have age spots, depending on your history of sun exposure.

Seasonal Variations: Winter, with its cold temperatures and dry air, can be a rough season for most mature skins. Flakiness, increased sensitivity, and chapping can occur. Spring and summer are when this skin type thrives, as added humidity means more moisture is available.

Cleansing: For the face, use a gentle, rich lotion or cream cleanser twice a day if you have dry skin or a water-based lotion if your skin is normal-to-oily. Carrot seed essential oil and rosehip seed base oil are highly regenerative and vitalizing and are good additions to your regular cleansing lotion or cream. Make sure to rinse well. For the body, use your favorite cleanser or gentle, natural soap.

Toning: Classic rosewater and glycerin, lavender, or German chamomile floral waters are excellent, gentle toners for facial skin.

Moisturizing: Depending upon the degree of dryness, a nutrient-rich, light- or medium-textured moisturizer that is easily absorbed is important for both the face and the body.

Special Treatments: A honey or moisturizing facial mask, used twice a week, hydrates the skin. An alpha- or beta-hydroxy acid treatment (depending upon your skin's sensitivity) used two to three times a week on both the face and the body will help refine the skin's surface and enhance absorption of your moisturizer. A fennel seed and lavender facial steam enjoyed once a week will hydrate and cleanse impurities from the pores. As desired, stimulate the circulation and increase blood flow with a facial massage using 2 to 3 drops of carrot seed essential oil mixed with 1 to 2 teaspoons (5–10 ml) of hazelnut oil. If necessary, an eye cream, applied nightly, will ease dryness in this delicate, thin-skinned area.

Sensitive Skin

Characteristics: Do you frequently react to many commonly used skin care products? Does your skin develop rashes, become irritated, blush quickly, overreact to sudden changes in temperature, and sunburn easily? Then it's probably sensitive. Sensitive skin can develop rosacea and couperose conditions (see chapter 6 for detailed descriptions).

All skin care products should be fragrance and color free and extremely gentle. Calendula-based products and German chamomile and lavender essential oils may be tolerated well by those of you with sensitive skin.

Seasonal Variations: This skin type tends to be normal-to-dry or very dry and thus winter's crisp, dry air can upset an already irritable complexion. Summer's heat, humidity, and strong sunlight can also wreak havoc, causing sunburn, blemishes, heat rashes, and ruddiness.

Cleansing: Gentle and nonabrasive are the key words here. A chamois facial cloth or a flannel washcloth are ideal to use as a cleansing tool. Avoid terry washcloths, tissues, or loofa pads. For the face, use a water-based lotion or cream cleanser twice a day. For the body, use your favorite cleanser or a gentle, natural soap. Make sure the product you choose does not strip your skin and cause it to feel dry and tight after cleansing.

Toning: Pure aloe vera gel or diluted with equal parts water, classic rose water and glycerin, or German chamomile floral water are generally nonirritating, soothing, and hydrating.

Moisturizing: A rapidly absorbing, light-to-medium weight moisturizer with good hydrating qualities will be most beneficial for this delicate skin on both the face and the body.

Special Treatments: Antioxidant facial gels, lotions, and creams can help nourish and desensitize this skin type. Keep a German chamomile or lavender floral water spray on hand to prevent dehydration and to soothe irritation. Very low concentrations of alpha- or beta-hydroxy acid can be used, if tolerated, once or twice per week on the face and the body to refine skin texture.

Environmentally Damaged Skin

Characteristics: Deep lines and wrinkles, hyperpigmentation (freckles and age spots), rough texture, and uneven skin tone are telltale signs of the life you've lead if you have this skin type. These characteristics can be the result of sun damage, pollution, climate, excessive living, and just plain neglect. Environmentally damaged skin ages prematurely. It's abused skin and it shows it! It can be oily, normal, or dry.

Seasonal Variations: Each season brings new challenges to environmentally damaged skin. Summer offers the chance for further sun abuse and winter weather makes it feel ultra-parched.

Care: A hydrating, moisturizing sunscreen should be worn every day to prevent further damage to an already abused skin.

Cleansing: For the face, a nonirritating, mild, water-based lotion or cream cleanser fortified with vitamins A, E, and C will deep clean and feed your skin — apply twice daily. A few drops of spike lavender, everlasting, lemongrass, or carrot seed essential oil added to your cleanser will help strengthen the dermal layer and encourage cell renewal. Cleanse your body with your favorite cleanser or gentle, natural soap.

Toning: A gentle, nondrying toner such as lavender floral water will refresh and remove any excess cleanser from the facial skin.

Moisturizing: A lotion or cream enhanced with rosehip seed oil will help to feed, rejuvenate, tone, and support cell membrane functions within the skin of both the face and the body.

Special Treatments: Regular exfoliation all over your body is important to combat the tendency toward flaky skin and uneven skin tone. Use an oatmeal scrub or an alpha- or beta-hydroxy acid treatment (depending upon your skin's sensitivity) twice a week as tolerated to refine skin and cleanse pores. Moisturizing eye creams are a necessity to help prevent this thin area from becoming like dried, crinkled parchment paper.

TOP TEN ENEMIES FOR ALL SKIN TYPES

1. Smoking. This nasty habit leads to puckering wrinkles around the mouth and fine squinty creases around your eyes. Smoking constricts blood vessels, restricts oxygen uptake, gives a gray color to your complexion, and literally eats up vitamin C, which is necessary for collagen formation.

2. Pollution. The solution to pollution is to avoid it whenever possible. If you live in a dirty, smoggy city and exercise out-of-doors, do so in the early morning when pollution concentration is at its lowest, otherwise, join a gym. Pollution affects your skin in the same way as smoking, minus the puckering and creasing.

3. Dry air. If you work in the typically dry air of a climate-controlled office or live in an arid climate, your skin can easily become parched and thirsty. Keep a hydrating floral water spray handy at all times.

4. Weight loss/gain. Your skin, though quite elastic, is not a rubber band. If you stretch anything too many times, it eventually loses its spring. Stretch marks and sagging, untoned skin can be the result of yo-yo dieting. Try to maintain a relatively constant weight.

5. Excessive pulling on the skin. Makeup and facial products should be applied using a gentle touch. A soft makeup sponge for color application and a light tapping or stroking motion when applying creams and lotions should be employed, otherwise you could encourage sagging.

6. Abusive exfoliation/overzealous cleansing. Washcloths and facial scrubs are designed to exfoliate your skin while cleansing. If you scrub your skin in the same manner used to remove the soap scum from your shower stall, you'll only irritate it and make matters worse, not better.

7. Alcohol. Consumption of alcoholic drinks, no matter how good they may make you feel (temporarily), have absolutely no place in a beautiful skin care regimen. Alcohol dehydrates you from the inside out, taxes your liver, and gobbles up your B vitamins.

8. Drugs. Check with your physician regarding the potential side effects of any medication you are taking. Some drugs may cause photosensitivity (sun sensitivity), dryness, blotchiness, or even mild acne.

9. Constipation. What goes in must exit — regularly! Toxins can build up within your body if your elimination is faulty, but they must eventually escape via some channel. Frequently the path of choice is your skin, so drink plenty of fresh water and eat lots of fiber to keep your plumbing running smoothly (and your skin looking smooth, too).

10. Sunlight. Excessive sun exposure leads to dry, wrinkled, leathery, blotchy, prematurely aged skin and possibly skin cancer. You need your daily dose of vitamin D. Fifteen minutes a day before 10:30 A.M. or after 4:30 P.M., when the sun's rays are not at their most intense, is my recommended daily allotment for sun exposure, without sunscreen. At other times of the day, always wear a sunscreen with an SPF of at least 15 to 25 to help prevent the signs of sun-damaged skin.

CHAPTER 4
The Salon and Spa Experience

Want to undo the damage of time, stress, environment, and neglect? Don't we all? Pay a visit to your local day spa or full-service salon and schedule an appointment with the resident esthetician. If you have the time, try to book at the very least a full deep-pore cleansing facial and back treatment. While the esthetician can't turn back the hands of time, she sure can take the edge off your nerves and rehydrate and deep cleanse your skin, leaving it smoother and more supple than when you arrived.

AN ESTHETICIAN'S TOUCH

Esthetics involves both creativity and psychology — it's not just about beauty, but also about instilling a feeling of well-being, health, and wholeness in the client. An esthetician's responsibilities to her clients include: assessing and meeting their emotional needs, understanding their physical wants and desires relating to skin care, and being able to make the client feel as if he or she is the most attractive and confident person alive. She accomplishes this by promoting clearer, smoother skin, providing a relaxing upper-body massage, artistically applying makeup, and giving her clients the pampering they need to feel good about themselves.

Since the vast majority of estheticians are female, I'm going to assume a bias toward the female gender when speaking of them. That is not to say that there aren't any trained male estheticians out there — it's just that in my experiences and at this time in the skin care world, they are few and far between.

Before entrusting your skin to another person's hands, you may want to ask some questions about the esthetician and the salon:

- Does the esthetician have a current license?
- Is she clean and well groomed, having short fingernails and hair that is up and out of the way?
- Is the salon neat and tidy? Does it have a professional setting?
- Is the treatment room tranquil and inviting?
- Are the esthetician's tools organized and new or sanitized? Is there a clean headwrap, towel, and robe for you?

BENEFITS OF PROFESSIONAL SKIN TREATMENT

- A complete analysis of skin type, and treatment recommendations
- A thorough, deep skin cleansing
- Increased blood circulation to the skin through steam and massage
- Focus on current skin disorders, with potential problems nipped in the bud
- Softened and hydrated skin
- Deep relaxation
- A self-esteem boost—you just plain look and feel better after a facial or body treatment!

PROFESSIONAL PAMPERING

Today's full-service salons and spas are a far cry from those of decades past. The better ones can be quite luxurious and plush, offering a complete sensory experience with myriad services including hairstyling, coloring, perming, straightening, manicuring and pedicuring, brow and lash tinting, facials, back treatments, herbal body wraps, the latest aromatherapy and anti-aging treatments, massage, body waxing, reflexology, and makeup application and instruction. More and more salons now also offer pre- and postsurgical skin care treatments and corrective makeup instruction.

There are several lush and lavish spas around the country that offer week-long packages of pure pampering with optional weight-loss, exercise, nutrition, and meditation counseling. If you've neither the money nor the time to get away for a week of beautification and purification, call your local salons and ask if they offer a day spa package that typically includes a haircut, blow-dry, manicure, pedicure, facial, makeup application, a pretty flower, and nourishing lunch. Salons and spas vary as to the services they offer and occasionally will customize their day-long experience to suit their patrons' personal needs.

WHAT TO EXPECT: SEVENTEEN STEPS TO RENEWED RADIANCE

To get the real scoop on the salon experience, I looked up an old friend, Donna Peri, who is the Head Esthetician at a wonderful day spa in Hyannis, Massachusetts. She was booked for five weeks solid! I promptly scheduled a facial, brow wax, and lash tint and informed her that she had to let me in on all the latest professional skin care secrets while she was giving me the works. I was about to embark on a relaxing and enlightening experience!

Most facials take, on average, 60 to 90 minutes, but Donna Peri decided to treat me to a two-and-a-half-hour escape from reality that left my skin with a rosy glow and my body tingling from head to toe. The following is a description of that wonderful treatment. Remember that salons vary in their procedures, and each esthetician follows her own special sequence and adds her own unique personality to the treatment.

SKINFORMATION

For skin fitness, Head Esthetician Donna Peri recommends a monthly or bi-monthly professional facial.

Prior to your facial, the esthetician will ask you to remove your shoes and clothing and slip into some type of fabric wrap that exposes your upper chest and shoulders. I was also given an organic cotton terrycloth robe and a pair of slippers to wear while I waited in the lounge area.

As I entered Donna's skin care room, the lighting was subtle, the air gently fragranced, the music soft and lyrical, and the mood tranquil. I removed my robe and slippers and reclined in her bodywork chair. She promptly covered me with a big, soft, warm blanket and tucked in my feet to avoid any chill.

Note: If, when you arrive for your facial, you are depressed or unduly stressed, alert your esthetician that you need a soothing and calming treatment, not one that may include potentially irritating products and procedures such as glycolic acid treatments, strong enzymes, or an extensive extraction session. When you are in a fragile state of mind, the last thing you need is to leave the salon with an aggravated complexion. You want to leave in a relaxed state of mind and body.

Step 1: Getting ready. Donna placed a cloth headwrap around my forehead to get my hair up and out of the way. She then moistened my face and throat with wonderfully soft cotton pads.

Step 2: Eye makeup removal. My eye makeup was removed using cotton pads soaked in a cool, soothing, chamomile and seaweed oil-based infusion.

Step 3: Cleansing. Her cleanser of choice was a mix of a gloriously scented honey and almond scrub combined with a seaweed-based cleanser. This produced a dual effect: cleansing and exfoliating, which was perfect for me as I have a slightly sensitive skin. Diluting the facial scrub with a creamy cleanser lessened the abrasiveness a straight facial scrub might have delivered. The delightful blend was gently swirled over my face and throat for about two minutes, then removed with the warm, damp cotton pads.

Step 4: Skin examination #1. Donna viewed my freshly cleansed skin through her illuminated magnifying glass and discovered a few rough dry spots, patches of built-up cellular debris. She applied a sloughing cream to smooth these areas that were apparently resistant to the mild exfoliating treatment I'd been given earlier.

Step 5: Massage preparation. My favorite part! My face, throat, chest, and shoulders were slathered with an intoxicatingly scented, neroli-rose, seaweed-based massage cream. It had the consistency of freshly-made buttercream frosting. A thick, moisturizing massage cream allows Donna to properly perform various facial and upper-body muscle manipulations. Her healing hands glide along the skin smoothly and evenly without any jerky motions.

The purpose of a massage is to induce a state of relaxation, to increase the blood supply to the skin, and to relax the follicles via increased perspiration and sebum secretion. Donna incorporates manual lymphatic drainage movements to alleviate puffiness around the eyes and the use of acupressure points to relieve muscle tension. Massage relaxes the facial muscles, which makes the skin more pliable. This enables the esthetician to remove impurities with ease. If you have acne, sunburned skin, or a couperose condition (sensitive skin characterized by dilated capillaries), your esthetician may choose not to perform a massage as this procedure could further irritate the condition.

Step 6: Steam and massage. Donna turned on her steam machine, or facial vaporizer, which delivered a fine, warm mist to my face and upper body from about 24 inches (60 cm) away. The purpose of receiving steam during your facial is to soften the dead surface skin cells so that they can easily be sloughed off during massage, to relax the follicle openings to aid in cleansing of deep-seated impurities, to temporarily increase blood circulation, and to hydrate the skin. I received a 45-minute simultaneous steam and upper body and facial massage! Much longer than the standard 10 to 15 minutes for this procedure, but we had a lot to catch up on and she could sense my high level of stress. Her soothing, well-trained fingers reached to the very core of my being. She calmed my frayed nerves, took the edge off my day, and

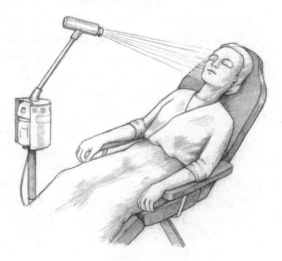

For maximum effect, a facial vaporizer should be stationed approximately 2 feet from your face.

We are born with two hungers — one is for food and the other is for touch. Touch is the first sense to develop inside the womb. And, of all the sensations we feel, touch is the most personally experienced. It is the sense most closely linked to the body's largest organ — the skin. Every inch of the skin is made for touching — and being touched. Therefore, the sense of touch — from birth until death — plays a tremendous role in human experience, and in the experience of being loved.

— *The Body Shop by Mail*, January 1998 issue

delivered a feel-good glow to my thirsty skin. My skin was so dehydrated, she had to reapply the massage cream three times!

Step 7: Massage cream removal. The steam is turned off and massage cream removed with cotton pads. At this point, I was practically asleep and felt like a limp noodle!

Step 8: Skin examination #2. After a few minutes of thorough investigation through her magnifying loop, Donna delivered her verdict: Normal skin, slightly dehydrated with mild clogging in the T-zone. You'd think that after all that massage cream and steam my skin would have recovered from its state of dehydration, but Donna informed me that it was still a bit thirsty. I simply wasn't using enough of the right moisturizer and I needed to increase my daily water intake.

Step 9: Extraction. Now came the fun part . . . extraction time. Anyone who's had a facial usually dreads these next few moments. Some estheticians are rough — poking, pinching, and prodding until your complexion looks like a war zone. There's actually an art to knowing how to properly pop a pimple or coax a blackhead from its hiding place. Thankfully Donna was very gentle. She'd prepared my skin properly through steam and massage so that any dirt, sebum, and lingering makeup in the clogged follicles was easily removed.

Step 10: High-frequency stimulation. A high-frequency machine, which looks like an electric toothbrush base topped by a mushroom-shaped glass wand, delivers a mild electric current when applied to the skin. The heat generated by this apparatus increases circulation and metabolic activity within the tissues. It's used after extraction procedures to destroy germs and bacteria and aid in healing of blemishes.

Donna moved the high-frequency wand in circular motions over my face and neck, concentrating on the T-zone where she performed the majority of my extractions.

Caution: If you are pregnant or you have a pacemaker, tell your esthetician prior to your facial. High-frequency current should not be used under these circumstances.

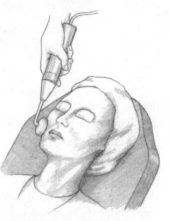

A high-frequency stimulation wand generates a mild electric current that kills germs and bacteria, aiding in healing blemishes.

Step 11: Toner application. My skin was freshened with an antiseptic lemon toner. Cool and tingly!

Step 12: Mineral mask application. A Dead Sea mud mineral mask was brushed onto my face, in extraction areas only, to calm, heal, and disinfect my skin.

Step 13: Waxing. My eyebrows were brushed into shape with an eyebrow brush and tamed by means of a small wax applicator that Donna used to roll on just enough warm wax to cover the strays hairs above and beneath my brows. She then laid a sliver of fabric over the wax, one area at a time, and gently rubbed her finger over it to help it adhere. Carefully and swiftly she pulled the fabric off in the opposite direction of the hair growth and immediately applied pressure with her hand to relieve the temporary sting. Ouch! It felt like an adhesive strip being quickly pulled off. The end result does look good, though! I shouldn't have to tweeze for another 4 weeks. Waxing removes the hair from beneath the skin, whereas shaving merely cuts it at the surface.

Donna then removed my mud mask with warm, damp cotton pads.

Step 14: Lash tinting. Jet black . . . that's the color I chose for my eyelashes. My lashes are dark brown with blond tips so they don't look as long as I'd like. Donna tinted them a glossy black. I treat myself to this luxury about once a year, usually around the holidays. I realize it's not a completely "natural" treatment, but performed properly, it's harmless, and it gives me quite an emotional and esthetic boost!

BUT IS IT NATURAL?

Facial and body waxing is a natural hair removal procedure preferred by many women — and some men — that leaves the skin very smooth, exfoliated, and hair-free for 3 to 4 weeks. If you use waxing as your exclusive method of hair removal over a period of several years, it tends to reduce hair growth density.

The depilatory wax product used by many salons is either 100 percent beeswax, a beeswax and paraffin blend, or a blend of resins and oils. A few salons may use a sugar-based product.

Caution: You should not undergo a waxing procedure if you are using the topical dermatological drugs Retin A or Accutane, or if you are using glycolic, alpha- or beta-hydroxy acids on your skin. These products dry and thin the outer layer of the epidermis, and waxing under those circumstances could cause severe irritation. Notify your esthetician if you are using any of these products.

Step 15: Hydrating mask. While the dye was setting, Donna applied a shea-butter hydrating mask to my face and neck. It smelled fabulous! The lash color was removed with wet cotton strips about 20 minutes later and the mask was removed with hot, damp towels.

Step 16: Vitamin C. Cool drops of topical vitamin C serum were ever so gently massaged into my skin to hydrate and nurture, to protect my skin from environmental assaults, and to help heal sun damage. The high-frequency machine was once again used, but this time to promote penetration of the vitamin C deep into the dermis where it can do the most good.

Step 17: Moisture sealant. A light, seaweed-based cream was pressed into my moist skin to seal in all the benefits I'd just received.

Result: My face practically glowed! It was plump, soft, rosy, and revitalized. The fine lines were gone and I'd swear I looked thirty instead of thirty-six. I'd been enlightened, educated, and best of all, I was completely calm. At peace with the world.

I'd recommend a facial to everyone, if not for the skin care benefits, for the relaxation alone. It is truly an incredible stress reducer.

PROFESSIONAL TIPS TO KEEP YOUR SKIN IN SUPER SHAPE

- Try to have a professional facial at least twice a year.
- Keep a mister bottle of either purified water or aromatic hydrosol handy at all times to refresh and hydrate your skin whenever you start to feel dry. This is especially important if you're a frequent flyer.
- Drink, drink, drink . . . at least eight glasses of purified water every day.
- Use sunscreen daily.
- Cleanse, tone, and moisturize twice a day with products specifically created for your skin type. As you get older, reevaluate your skin type. Everything changes with age!
- Eat a healthy diet and get plenty of exercise.
- Learn to manage the stress in your life. Stress wreaks havoc on even the most beautiful skin.

CHAPTER 5
Ingredients, Tools, and Supplies for Making and Storing Natural Skin Care Treatments

This chapter is a descriptive journey through my "green world." I use all of the natural ingredients that follow in the personal care products I make for myself and my friends, family, and clients. By adopting at least a few of these ingredients into your skin care repertoire, you will be educating yourself about what you put in and on your body. Only you can take control of your skin's health!

BASE OILS

Base oils are derived from nuts, seeds, vegetables, and fruits. They have mild therapeutic properties, but as the name implies, they are most often used as a base or carrier oil to which essential oils and herbs are added when making oils, lotions, or creams.

The best oils to purchase for skin care purposes are cold- or expeller-pressed, as they are not extracted at extremely high temperatures and/or with a chemical solvent. (Exposure to high temperatures and chemical solvents can destroy natural flavors, aromas, antioxidant properties, and beneficial trace minerals and vitamins.) Cold-pressed oils are processed at a relatively low temperature (150–250°F, or 65–120°C). Expeller-pressed oils have been mechanically pressed from the nut, seed, fruit, or vegetable from which it is derived. Cold- and expeller-pressed oils, by the way, are also highly recommended for use in cooking and salad dressings, as they have a better flavor and higher nutritional value than conventionally processed oils.

Base oils, with the exception of avocado, hazelnut, jojoba, and extra-virgin olive, tend to become rancid if stored at room temperature for

PRESERVATION

To prolong the shelf life of your base oil, pierce eight to ten vitamin E capsules. Add the contents of the capsules to every 8 ounces of oil.

more than 4 to 6 months; they should be refrigerated. The oils described below should have only a trace of fragrance, if any at all. If the oil has a strong or "off" smell (with the exception of olive oil), then it's probably old. Purchase base oils through reputable mail-order suppliers (see resources) or better health food stores with a high inventory turnover. Don't hesitate to return the product if it is bad.

ALMOND OIL

Description: A clear to very pale yellow oil pressed from sweet almond seeds (kernels). Full of vitamins and minerals. Reasonably priced and widely available.

Uses: From massage oils to lotions, creams to masks, almond oil is good for all skin types, especially dry, inflamed, or itchy skin. A first-rate, all-purpose oil.

AVOCADO OIL

Description: A clear, medium to dark green oil derived from the fatty fruit pulp. Rich in protein, vitamins, and fatty acids. A very stable oil with a long shelf life. Moderately priced and sometimes difficult to find.

Uses: Especially good blended with other base oils and used as an after-bath body or facial oil — use 1 part avocado oil to 10 parts other base oils. The perfect, nourishing oil for dull, lifeless, dry, and devitalized skin; eczema; and psoriasis.

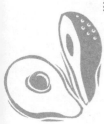

BORAGE SEED OIL

Description: A pale yellow oil pressed from the seeds. Very rich in beneficial GLA (gamma linolenic acid), vitamins, and minerals. Expensive, but worth it.

Uses: Taken internally, borage seed oil lessens PMS symptoms and helps to lubricate joints and skin. When blended with avocado, jojoba, hazelnut, or almond oil, it is used externally to treat eczema, psoriasis, and signs of premature aging. Dilute with other base oils using a 1 to 10 ratio.

CASTOR OIL

Description: A very thick, clear to slightly yellow oil processed from the seeds of an annual shrub. Extremely moisturizing. Inexpensive and easy to find.

Uses: I like it for the staying power and shine it provides to my lip balm and gloss recipes. Particularly good for softening rough, dry heels, knees, elbows, and patches of eczema and psoriasis.

COCONUT PALM OIL

Description: Expressed from coconut meat or flesh, this white semisolid fat melts at room temperature. Widely available and inexpensive.

Uses: Excellent as a massage or bath oil or when used in lotions and creams. A mild, gentle oil, good for sensitive and infant skin.

HAZELNUT OIL

Description: A clear, pale yellow oil derived from the pressed kernel, hazelnut oil has a mild, nutty fragrance. High in vitamin E and fatty acids. It has a light, penetrating quality that makes it good for all skin types. Usually only available through mail-order suppliers, moderately priced.

Uses: One of the best base oils used in face creams and lotions because of its lightness and stability (it is not prone to rancidity). Especially good for aging skin.

JOJOBA OIL

Description: Actually a liquid plant wax, this clear, yellow oil is pressed from the seeds. The thick oil closely resembles human sebum in consistency. Will not become rancid; hardens in cold weather. Expensive, but relatively easy to find.

Uses: Good for inflamed skin, eczema, psoriasis, rough or dry skin, and acne. Penetrates easily and is very compatible with human skin.

OLIVE OIL

Description: A clear green oil with a strong olive fragrance taken from the first pressing of ripe olives. High in vitamin E. Moderately priced, widely available. Be sure to choose the extra-virgin variety.

Uses: Though a very high-quality cosmetic oil, I rarely use it, except when combining with salt to make body scrubs or salves, because of its overpowering fragrance and color.

ROSEHIP SEED OIL

Description: Clear, reddish in color, derived from the seeds of the ripened fruit of *Rosa rubiginosa* (commonly known as Rosa Mosqueta). Extremely high in essential fatty acids. Expensive and usually only available from better health food stores or mail-order suppliers.

Uses: Used with much success in treatments for skin damage that has resulted in premature aging, dehydration, wrinkles, or scars. Highly recommended for mature, dry, and sun-damaged skin.

Contraindication: Should not be used on skin that is oily or acneic.

SESAME OIL

Description: Derived from the pressed seeds, this clear, golden oil is rich in vitamins A and E and protein. It's a very stable base oil, meaning that it has a long shelf life.

Uses: Used in sunscreens, salves, and lotions. Superb as a body oil for normal-to-dry skin.

Note: Do not use the toasted varieties of sesame oil in your skin care products.

SOYBEAN OIL

Description: A clear, yellow, highly refined, widely available, inexpensive oil. Commonly found in grocery stores under the label of "vegetable oil." Check the ingredients panel and it should read "100 percent soybean oil."

Uses: A terrific massage oil. Penetrates readily with no greasy residue. Not my number one choice, though, because of the chemical residues found in most brands as a result of processing, but can be used in a pinch. Try to find an organically produced soybean oil.

ESSENTIAL OILS

Essential oils are steam distilled from flowers, roots, barks, seeds, leaves, resins, or twigs, or are pressed from citrus rinds. Unlike a vegetable or nut oil, an essential oil is not actually an "oil" because it does not contain fatty acids and is not prone to rancidity. For extraction purposes, low pressure and low temperature methods ensure top-quality fragrance and therapeutic value. I purchase my essential oils from a handful of companies I've come to know and trust (see resources). Their oils are of superior quality and suitable for aromatherapeutic skin care treatments. Many health food stores and herb shops also carry quality essential oils.

An essential oil is the life-force or the "soul" of the plant. Each precious, aromatic, highly volatile, concentrated drop of an essential oil contains plant hormones and organic chemical compounds that regenerate and oxygenate the skin. They are important to include in therapeutic skin care treatments because their small molecular structure allows them to easily penetrate into the dermis to nourish, rejuvenate, and regenerate skin cells. Unlike most ingredients in a moisturizing cream, which stay primarily on the skin's surface, essential oils are absorbed all the way down to the subcutaneous tissue layer.

ESSENTIAL OIL PRECAUTIONS

Essential oils are highly concentrated natural products and must be used with caution. To test for potential allergic reactions, try this patch test: Combine 1 or 2 drops of the essential oil in question with 1 teaspoon (5 ml) base oil in a small bowl. Apply a dab on the underside of your wrist, inside your upper arm, behind your ear, or behind your knee, and wait 12 to 24 hours. If no irritation develops, it is generally safe to use that particular oil.

BLUE CYPRESS (CALLITRIS INTRATROPICA)
Description: Distilled from the branches and leaves of an Australian tree — very rare, but exceptional! The oil is clear, medium blue-green in color, and smells like musty, wet, forest-floor leaves, but when applied to warm skin develops a mellow, sandalwood-like fragrance. Quite wonderful, really!

Cosmetic Properties and Uses: Superior essential oil for dry or mature skin. Contains antiviral properties. Can be used as an effective replacement for essential oil of sandalwood, which is rapidly becoming endangered. Excellent treatment for ridding your skin of warts.

CALENDULA *(CALENDULA OFFICINALIS)*
Description: Derived from the petals of the beautiful orange or yellow flower. The oil is clear, deep orange in color and has a heavy, intoxicating, herbal fragrance.
Cosmetic Properties and Uses: Antiseptic, antifungal, and anti-inflammatory. Good for healing scar tissue, burns, bruises, acne, insect bites, and cuts. Gentle enough for young children. I normally add a few drops to every cosmetic I make or purchase. One of my favorites!

CARROT SEED *(DAUCUS CAROTA)*
Description: Distilled from carrot seeds, this essential oil is clear, yellowish-orange in color, and smells slightly spicy-sweet, reminiscent of fresh carrots.
Cosmetic Properties and Uses: High in beta-carotene. A very nourishing, vitalizing, and restorative oil. Stimulates skin elasticity. Good for all skin types, especially wrinkled, normal-to-dry, and sagging skin.
Contraindication: Should not be used by epileptics or women who are pregnant.

CHAMOMILE, GERMAN *(MATRICARIA RECUTITA)*
Common Names: Blue chamomile, wild chamomile
Description: An intensely deep blue oil, distilled from the flowers of this lacy, delicate, pretty plant. The heavy chamomile fragrance tends to overpower any formula it is added to and the blue color also dominates, turning many cosmetics blue-green.
Cosmetic Properties and Uses: High in azulene content. Extremely soothing and healing to irritated, couperose, normal-to-dry, and sensitive skin. A strong anti-inflammatory and antifungal natural medicine. Powerful relaxant. Beneficial for acne when blended with spike lavender and everlasting essential oils.

EUCALYPTUS (EUCALYPTUS DIVES)

Common Name: Blue peppermint eucalyptus

Description: A clear, pale yellow-to-green oil with a refreshing menthol/balsam/camphor-like fragrance. It is distilled from the leaves of this plant.

Cosmetic Properties and Uses: Recommended in formulas for balancing the production of excess sebum in oily or acneic skin. Used as an inhalant to relieve chest congestion.

Contraindication: Should not be used by epileptics or women who are pregnant.

GERANIUM, ROSE (PELARGONIUM X ASPERUM, GRAVEOLENS)

Description: A clear, pale greenish-yellow oil distilled from the leaves of this beautiful plant. Has a strong, earthy, minty-sweet, uplifting, almost roselike aroma.

Cosmetic Properties and Uses: Good for normal and normal-to-oily skin. Has mild astringent properties. Helps to heal burns, abrasions, ulcers, and acne when combined with spike lavender and rosemary.

EVERLASTING or IMMORTELLE (HELICHRYSUM ITALICUM)

Description: A clear, yellowish oil distilled from the whole plant. Highly aromatic with a currylike smell.

Cosmetic Properties and Uses: Very strong anti-inflammatory, antibacterial, and antifungal. Said to be even more potent than German chamomile. Indicated for healing bruises, open wounds and cuts, varicose veins, acne, eczema, and psoriasis. Very soothing. Stimulates new cell formation.

INULA (INULA GRAVEOLENS)

Description: A clear-to-pale green oil distilled from the flowers with a medicinal, sweet, camphorlike aroma.

Cosmetic Properties and Uses: Ideal for oily, acneic, overly clogged skin. Loosens sebum. Highly antibacterial and mucolytic. Works well blended with eucalyptus and spike lavender.

Contraindication: Should not be used by epileptics or women who are pregnant.

BUYER BE AWARE

Essential oil production is a labor-intensive and material-expensive project. It takes approximately 500 pounds of rosemary to produce 1 pound of oil. Jasmine absolute, one of the most expensive essential oils (retails for three to six hundred dollars per ounce), requires approximately eight million hand-picked blossoms, harvested before sunrise, to produce just over 2 pounds of oil. A high-quality oil is expensive, but it is worth it. Unfortunately, there are some pretty low-quality oils out there, so you need to know the distinguishing features of a quality essential oil.

1. Look for "g & a" (genuine and authentic), "vintage," or "organic" on the label, or ask for therapeutic or pharmaceutical grade oils. These essential oils have been steam distilled at low temperatures. You will pay more for this type of processing, but you'll be ensured of a pure, effective product.

2. Essential oils are highly volatile and will evaporate quickly. Place a drop or two of essential oil on a sheet of plain paper, spread it around a bit, and leave it alone for 5 to 10 hours. A real essential oil will evaporate and will not leave a stain, or perhaps a very minor one. A vegetable oil will leave a greasy stain, as potato chips do if placed in a brown paper bag.

3. Vegetable oils have a greasy feel; essential oils do not. Rub a little vegetable oil between your fingers and notice how slippery it is. Now rub a drop of essential oil between the fingers of your other hand. It may initially feel greasy, but the essential oil will quickly be absorbed or feel more like water. If the essential oil feels like vegetable oil, it probably has been diluted.

JUNIPER BERRY (JUNIPERUS COMMUNIS)

Description: A clear, pale yellow oil distilled from the berries or small branches of this evergreen shrub. Has a sweet balsam, woody fragrance.

Cosmetic Properties and Uses: A good antiseptic and cleansing addition to products for oily skin or eczema. Is frequently used in massage oil formulas for cellulite because of its strong diuretic action.

Contraindication: Avoid if you have a history of kidney problems, are pregnant, or are epileptic.

LAVENDER (LAVANDULA ANGUSTIFOLIA)

Description: A clear, yellow-green oil steam-distilled from the fragrant blossoms. Highly valued as a potent healing agent and floral perfume additive.

Cosmetic Properties and Uses: Good for all skin types. One of the few oils that can be used "neat," or undiluted. Powerful relaxant and a strong yet gentle antiseptic; effective as a remedy for sunburn, bee stings, muscle cramps, burns, and insomnia. Safe for everyone, including infants and pregnant women.

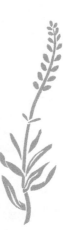

LEMONGRASS (CYMBOPOGON CITRATUS)

Description: A clear, yellowish brown liquid distilled from the grassy leaves of this plant. Has a pleasant lemony fragrance.

Cosmetic Properties and Uses: Used in cleansers and moisturizers for normal-to-oily skin because of its mild astringent property. Also good for sagging, devitalized smoker's skin — helps to eliminate wastes.

Contraindication: Do not use on sensitive or irritated skin.

ORANGE, SWEET (CITRUS SINENSIS)

Description: A clear, pale-to-vibrant orange oil with a strong, fruity, uplifting, orangelike fragrance. Extracted from the pressed fruit rind.

Cosmetic Properties and Uses: Recommended for all skin types except very dry. Slightly astringent.

Contraindication: Can cause skin to become photosensitive (abnormally reactive to sunlight). Do not use if you are pregnant or epileptic.

OREGANO *(ORIGANUM COMPACTUM, O. VULGARE)*

Description: Distilled from the leaves and stems of these highly aromatic members of the mint family. It has an oregano/mint fragrance. Very warming on the skin with a clear, yellow to earthy brown color.

Cosmetic Properties and Uses: Powerful antiseptic and antiviral. Good for treating warts, insect bites, fungal infections, and general skin infections.

Contraindication: This essential oil is a skin irritant and must be well diluted. Avoid if you are pregnant or epileptic.

PEPPERMINT MITCHAM *(MENTHA X PIPERITA)*

Description: A clear-to-pale green oil distilled from the stems and leaves. This particular type of peppermint essential oil has a very sweet, almost candylike aroma, without the sharp bite that other peppermints have. If "Mitcham" is unavailable, regular peppermint is fine. Mitcham just happens to be my personal favorite.

Cosmetic Properties and Uses: Very refreshing, cooling, and astringent when made into a facial toner or body splash or cleanser for normal-to-oily skin. An excellent antiseptic when blended with tea tree and orange essential oils.

Contraindication: A potential skin irritant if used in large amounts. Do not use if you are pregnant or epileptic.

ESSENTIAL OIL STORAGE TIPS

◆ Because essential oils can be harmful if ingested, it is important to store them out of reach of children and pets.

◆ To prolong the shelf life of an essential oil, do not store the oil in a bottle with a rubber top. The strong vapors emitting from the oil will gradually weaken the rubber and allow air to enter the bottle, and the precious volatile healing properties will evaporate prematurely. If you intend to keep a particular bottle of oil longer than 60 months, seal it with a plastic screw-top cap and reserve the dropper for that essential oil only.

ROSEMARY (*ROSMARINUS OFFICINALIS,* CHEMOTYPE VERBENON)

Description: This oil is a colorless, clear liquid. Has an earthy, strong fragrance with a dominant camphor/eucalyptus note. Distilled from the stems and leaves of this plant.

Cosmetic Properties and Uses: Known for stimulating new cell formation. Can benefit all skin types, and particularly good in regenerative, nurturing skin care formulations for wrinkled, devitalized, aging, acneic, burned, scarred, or sun-damaged skin.

Contraindication: Do not use if you are pregnant or suffer from epilepsy or high blood pressure.

SPIKE LAVENDER (*LAVANDULA SPICA*)

Description: A clear, pale yellowish green oil distilled from the flowers. Highly aromatic, floral, with a clean, classic lavender fragrance.

Cosmetic Properties and Uses: Helps to normalize and balance the skin. Good for all skin types. Also an effective antiseptic for burns, cuts, and insect bites. Makes a nice addition to a relaxing massage oil formula.

Contraindication: Avoid during pregnancy or if you suffer from epilepsy.

TEA TREE (*MELALEUCA ALTERNIFOLIA*)

Description: A clear, pale yellow oil that is distilled from the leaves of an Australian tree. Has a pungent, balsam/camphor medicinal scent.

Cosmetic Properties and Uses: Powerful antibacterial, antifungal, and antiseptic. Helps heal acne, open wounds, cuts, ulcers, and infections. Makes a good addition to cleansers for acneic skin.

THYME (*THYMUS VULGARIS,* CHEMOTYPE LINALOL)

Description: A clear-to-yellowish oil with less "bite" than other, hotter thyme oils, this is a softer, nonirritating variety of thyme. Distilled from the branches, leaves, and flowers. Has a sweet/spicy, fresh scent.

Cosmetic Properties and Uses: A strong antiseptic. Highly recommended in treatments for infectious skin diseases.

Very healing for oozing acne and rashes resulting from poison oak, ivy, sumac, or general contact dermatitis. **Contraindication:** Do not use during pregnancy or if you suffer from high blood pressure or epilepsy.

WHAT'S A CHEMOTYPE?

Plants of the same botanical species can produce essential oils of distinctly different compositions, or chemotypes. The reason for this is not completely understood, but factors such as where the plant is grown and its genetic lineage can contribute to this phenomenon, known as *chemical polymorphism*.

For example, as you can see under the listing for rosemary, the botanical Latin identification is followed by a chemotype identification, specifically verbenon. This is the chemical component, or chemotype, most characteristic for that species of plant. I've chosen the verbenon chemotype because it is a very gentle, nonirritating essential oil that is a staple for high-quality skin care preparations.

Only the labels of superior quality, pharmaceutical or aromatherapeutic grade essential oils will offer these chemotype distinctions. Try to locate these specific types of essential oils so that you can achieve maximum results with your homemade preparations.

— Adapted from *Aromatherapy Course, Part I, Essential Oils,* 2nd edition, by Dr. Kurt Schnaubelt

FLORAL WATERS

Floral waters, or aromatic hydrosols, are a pure, natural by-product of the essential oil distillation process. These fragrant waters are saturated with the water-soluble compounds present in the plants and are gentle enough to use when an essential oil would be too strong or would be irritating to a particular skin type or condition.

Hydrosols make wonderful toners, splashes, and sprays that are soothing, hydrating, lightly moisturizing, and mildly antiseptic. Additionally, floral waters can replace distilled plain water in a cream or lotion recipe to increase the therapeutic value and fragrance. They can be purchased in better health food stores and herb shops or from the mail-order companies listed in the resource section.

CHAMOMILE, GERMAN (*MATRICARIA RECUTITA*)

Cosmetic Properties and Uses: Soothing and balancing, good for all skin types, especially sensitive, irritated, and couperose. Powerful anti-inflammatory with a haunting floral, intoxicating, relaxing fragrance.

LAVENDER (*LAVANDULA* SPP.)

Cosmetic Properties and Uses: This classic water has a clean, floral fragrance. Its gentle antiseptic, calming, and healing qualities bring relief to skin irritations and sunburn. An ideal toner for normal or dry skin.

NEROLI or ORANGE BLOSSOM (*CITRUS AURANTIUM*)

Cosmetic Properties and Uses: Sweet, orange/floral fragrance from the flowers of the bitter orange. Acts as a mild, refreshing astringent. Beneficial to acneic, irritated, oily, and sensitive skin.

ROSE OTTO (*ROSA DAMASCENA*)

Cosmetic Properties and Uses: Wonderfully rich, romantic, old-fashioned floral fragrance. Balancing, calming, and mildly astringent. Helps revive tired, devitalized skin and eyes; gentle enough to be used directly on the eyes.

> *May your life be like a wildflower, growing freely in the beauty and joy of each day.*
>
> — Native American proverb

FRUITS

The following is a list of my favorite fruits to use in natural skin care recipes. These fruits contain fruit acids, also called alpha-hydroxy acids (AHAs) or beta-hydroxy agents (BHAs), that are extremely good for the skin when applied externally. AHAs dissolve the bond that holds dead skin cells together and increases hydration while BHAs naturally dissolve dry, flaky surface skin and stimulate cell renewal. All skin types from oily to very dry can benefit from these remarkably effective and inexpensive fruit acids.

When purchasing, try to find organically grown fruit. *Note:* For maximum skin rejuvenation, all fruits should be used in their raw state.

APPLE (AHA)

Parts Used: Pulp, freshly pressed juice
Cosmetic Properties and Uses: Contains malic acid. Acts as a mild astringent. Soothing for sensitive and acneic skin. Mixed with white cosmetic clay, makes a gentle, exfoliating mask.

BANANA (AHA)

Parts Used: Pulp
Cosmetic Properties and Uses: Nourishing and moisturizing. Extremely gentle. Recommended for normal and dry skin. Can be used straight as a mask or blended with white cosmetic clay for added exfoliation and tightening.

BLACKBERRY AND RASPBERRY (AHA)

Parts Used: Freshly pressed, strained juice
Cosmetic Properties and Uses: Contains lactic acid. Can be applied with a cotton ball directly to all but the most sensitive or sunburned skin as an exfoliating tonic and then rinsed off. Moderately astringent.

CITRUS FRUITS — GRAPEFRUIT, LEMON, LIME, ORANGE, TANGERINE (AHA)

Parts Used: Freshly pressed juice, rind (zest)

Cosmetic Properties and Uses: Contains citric acid. Astringent and fragrant. Good for oily and normal skin. Juice and zest can be added to toners, spritzers, masks, and lotions.

Contraindication: Not recommended for sensitive or inflamed skin.

GRAPE (AHA)

Parts Used: Freshly pressed juice

Cosmetic Properties and Uses: Contains tartaric acid. Apply juice to face with cotton ball to help improve skin texture, rinse. Safe for all skin types.

PAPAYA (BHA)

Parts Used: Pulp

Cosmetic Properties and Uses: Contains the enzyme papain. Applied as a wet mask, will help to even out skin tone and soften skin. Especially useful for a fading tan or dry, flaky, rough skin.

Contraindication: May be irritating to sensitive, sunburned, or inflamed skin.

PINEAPPLE (BHA)

Parts Used: Freshly pressed juice

Cosmetic Properties and Uses: Contains the enzyme bromelain. Will dissolve dead, dry skin cells resulting in smoother skin.

Contraindication: May be irritating to sensitive, sunburned, or inflamed skin.

STRAWBERRY (AHA)

Parts Used: Pulp

Cosmetic Properties and Uses: Acts as a gentle astringent. Safe for all skin types. Pulp may be thickened with white cosmetic clay and applied as an exfoliating mask.

GRAINS, NUTS, AND SEEDS

I always have a generous supply of the following four "skin foods" in my kitchen. They are staples for the kitchen cosmetologist. All ingredients should be organically grown, if possible, and used in raw form. To ensure freshness, nuts and seeds should be kept in the freezer. Oatmeal can be stored in a cool, dry cabinet.

ALMOND

Forms Used: Ground almonds (almond meal)
Cosmetic Properties and Uses: High in skin-loving nutrients and fat. Used as a facial and body scrub base to gently exfoliate rough, dry skin.

FLAXSEED

Forms Used: Ground seeds (flaxseed meal) or cracked seeds
Cosmetic Properties and Uses: When water is added to the whole, cracked seeds or meal, the resulting emollient gel can be strained and massaged into the skin to soothe, nourish, and help heal minor irritations, acne, and sunburn.

OATMEAL

Forms Used: Ground oatmeal
Cosmetic Properties and Uses: Added to bath water, oatmeal relieves itchy, rashy skin and allergic reactions from poison ivy, oak, and sumac or insect bites. Ground oatmeal can also be used as a mask base for all skin types and as a gentle facial scrub for sensitive or couperose skin.

SUNFLOWER

Forms Used: Ground seeds (sunflower seed meal)
Cosmetic Properties and Uses: Very rich in fatty acids, emollients, and beneficial nutrients. Meal makes a gentle, moisturizing scrub and mask base for normal-to-dry skin.

MAKING GRAIN, SEED, AND NUT MEALS

Almond Meal: To make ½ cup (125 ml) almond meal, grind (in 10-second pulses) approximately 50 large, raw almonds in a blender, coffee grinder, or food processor until the consistency is that of finely grated Parmesan cheese. Due to their high fat content, it's very easy to overblend almonds and end up with almond butter, especially if you use a small grinder that generates lots of heat. This is actually not a bad thing, as it is quite tasty and can be used just like peanut butter, but it's not the result you're after!

Flaxseed Meal: To make ½ cup (125 ml) flaxseed meal, blend a heaping ½ cup (125 ml) seeds in a blender, coffee grinder, or food processor until the consistency is that of coarse whole wheat flour.

Ground Oatmeal: To make ½ cup (125 ml) ground oatmeal, blend ¾ to 1 cup (180 to 250 ml) of regular or old-fashioned oats in a blender, coffee grinder, or food processor until the consistency is that of fine flour.

Sunflower Seed Meal: To make ½ cup (125 ml) sunflower seed meal, grind ¾ cup (180 ml) of large seeds (hulled) in a blender, coffee grinder, or food processor until the consistency is that of finely grated Parmesan cheese.

HERBS, SPICES, AND FLOWERS

Herbs have been used for thousands of years by every culture for their medicinal, fragrant, and skin-pampering qualities. The following are my favorite herbs for skin care. They are easily found in most health food stores, herb shops, or through mail-order suppliers (see resources). Try to purchase organically grown herbs if possible, or grow your own. Fresh is always best!

ALOE VERA *(ALOE VERA)*

Parts Used: Gel or juice from the leaves
Cosmetic Properties and Uses: The gel and juice helps heal all types of burns, insect bites, and rashes. Slightly astringent and very soothing. Terrific when mixed with a drop or two of lavender essential oil and sprayed on sunburned skin.

GEL OR JUICE?

Aloe vera gel can be lumpy at times. If you're making a preparation to be spritzed on your face or body, you'll probably prefer to work with aloe vera juice. You can either purchase the juice or make it yourself at home: Mix ¼ cup (60 ml) of the gel with 1 tablespoon (15 ml) distilled water and blend for 15 seconds.

CALENDULA *(CALENDULA OFFICINALIS)*

Common Name: Pot marigold
Parts Used: Flower petals
Cosmetic Properties and Uses: Contains antifungal, anti-inflamitory, antiseptic, and antibacterial properties. As an infused oil, calendula is healing to cuts, bruises, rashes, and irritated skin when combined with spike lavender, tea tree, German chamomile, or thyme essential oil.

CHAMOMILE, GERMAN *(MATRICARIA RECUTITA)*

Common Names: Blue chamomile, wild chamomile
Parts Used: Flowering tops
Cosmetic Properties and Uses: Cooled tea is a good anti-inflammatory treatment for pimples and acne, and the dried, ground flowers are a good addition to gentle facial scrubs. The whole, fresh flowers can be added to bath water for a relaxing, fragrant, skin-pampering way to end your day.

CINNAMON *(CINNAMOMUM AROMATICUM)*

Common Name: Cassia
Parts Used: Powdered inner bark

Cosmetic Properties and Uses: Mildly astringent, antiseptic, and fragrant. In combination with powdered, dried chamomile flowers, white cosmetic clay, and ground oatmeal, makes a gentle exfoliating scrub or mask.

COMFREY *(SYMPHYTUM OFFICINALE)*
Parts Used: Leaves, root
Cosmetic Properties and Uses: High in minerals, protein, and allantoin. Mildly astringent, emollient, mucilaginous. Tea made from chopped root is healing, skin-nurturing, and speeds cell renewal. A compress can be applied to cuts, burns, eczema, and psoriasis to bring quick relief to inflammation, swelling, and irritation.

ELDERFLOWER *(SAMBUCUS CANADENSIS)*
Parts Used: Flowers
Cosmetic Properties and Uses: The fragrant flowers make a soothing wash for both eye and skin irritations. Good for all skin types.

EYEBRIGHT *(EUPHRASIA ROSTKOVIANA)*
Parts Used: Flowers, stems, and leaves
Cosmetic Properties and Uses: The entire plant is used to make an infusion that soothes irritated, strained eyes. Mildly astringent, antiseptic, and anti-inflammatory.

FENNEL *(FOENICULUM VULGARE)*
Parts Used: Seeds
Cosmetic Properties and Uses: The fragrant, licorice-scented seeds, when added to boiling water, make a deep cleansing facial steam that is especially good for normal-to-dry and wrinkled skin. The tea can be used as a healing tonic for chapped skin.

LAVENDER (*LAVANDULA* SPP.)
Parts Used: Flowers, leaves
Cosmetic Properties and Uses: Can be used as an infusion as a soothing facial wash for all skin types, especially irritated and acneic skin.

HERB STORAGE TIP

Dried herbs should be stored in dark-colored glass jars, tins, or zip-seal plastic bags, in a dark, cool, dry place. A good-quality herb will keep for up to one year.

Ground, dried flowers can be combined with ground oatmeal and used as a calming, gentle facial scrub and mask for even the most sensitive skins.

LEMON BALM *(MELISSA OFFICINALIS)*
Parts Used: Leaves, stems
Cosmetic Properties and Uses: Refreshing lemony fragrance and flavor. The tea is an excellent addition to light lotions and creams to help heal and cleanse skin affected by pimples, acne, insect bites, and rashes. Lemon balm infusion has antiviral properties, which is good for your irritated skin, harmful for pesky bacteria. Combined with vinegar, this herb makes a lovely facial rinse that can be used to balance your skin's pH after cleansing.

LEMONGRASS *(CYMBOPOGON CITRATUS)*
Parts Used: Leaf blades
Cosmetic Properties and Uses: Has a refreshing, lemony fragrance. As a tea, makes an excellent antiseptic for oily skin. Acts as an astringent cleansing agent in facials steams and toners.

LICORICE *(GLYCYRRHIZA GLABRA)*
Parts Used: Roots
Cosmetic Properties and Uses: Helps reduce skin inflammation resulting from allergies or rashes. Especially good used in acne treatments and poison plant rashes. Soothing and healing.

HOW TO MAKE AN HERBAL INFUSION

Herbal infusions, teas, or waters are frequently used as an ingredient in splashes, tonics, lotions, creams, and bath additives. To make, pour 1 cup (250 ml) of boiling water over 1 teaspoon (5 ml) dried herb or 2 teaspoons (10 ml) fresh herb. Cover, steep 5 to 10 minutes, and strain. Cool and use as directed.

MARSH MALLOW (ALTHAEA OFFICINALIS)

Parts Used: Roots

Cosmetic Properties and Uses: The Greek word *althaea* means "to heal." Roots contain a soothing mucilage and when steeped in simmering water produce a "healing goo" that is quite beneficial for weather-beaten, chapped, or sun-damaged skin. An excellent anti-inflammatory when applied to acneic skin.

PEPPERMINT (MENTHA X PIPERITA)

Parts Used: Leaves, stems

Cosmetic Properties and Uses: Stimulating, refreshing, antiseptic, fragrant, and antiviral. Peppermint vinegar balances the skin's pH after cleansing. Peppermint infusion is cooling to hot, sweaty "summer skin" and has a mild, astringent quality that helps to remove excess oil.

RED CLOVER (TRIFOLIUM PRATENSE)

Parts Used: Flowers

Cosmetic Properties and Uses: Often considered a weed, the reddish pink blossoms of this plant are used as an anti-inflammatory, calming, and cleansing ingredient in products for normal-to-dry skin. They're a wonderful addition in facial steam blends for dry, irritated skin.

ROSE (ROSA SPP.)

Parts Used: Petals

Cosmetic Properties and Uses: I use the dried, ground petals mixed with white cosmetic clay and ground oatmeal to make a gentle facial exfoliant and mask that can be used by all skin types.

ROSEMARY (ROSMARINUS OFFICINALIS)

Parts Used: Leaves

Cosmetic Properties and Uses: An infusion made from the aromatic and antiseptic leaves can be used by all skin types as a facial or body splash, or added to lotions and cream recipes in place of distilled water. Also beneficial in facial steams to help cleanse the pores.

SAGE *(SALVIA OFFICINALIS)*
Parts Used: Leaves, flowers
Cosmetic Properties and Uses: A strongly fragrant infusion made from the astringent and antiseptic leaves is an effective cleanser for normal-to-oily skin. A cup of sage vinegar added to your bath will help relieve itchiness caused by heat rash or poison ivy, oak, or sumac.

THYME *(THYMUS VULGARIS)*
Parts Used: Leaves
Cosmetic Properties and Uses: Disinfectant and antiseptic. Thyme infusion is a good wash for cuts, scrapes, ulcers, and acne. Recommended for normal-to-oily skin. Try to grow a patch in your garden so that you can make fresh thyme vinegar to freshen your skin and also to put in your salad dressing — yum!

YARROW *(ACHILLEA MILLEFOLIUM)*
Parts Used: Leaves, flowers
Cosmetic Properties and Uses: Very strong astringent. A poultice of the crushed, fresh leaves applied to cuts arrests bleeding. A flower infusion can be used to treat eczema and acne.

HOW TO DO A PATCH TEST WITH HERBS

In a small bowl, combine ½ teaspoon (2.5 ml) fresh or dried chopped herb in question with 1 teaspoon (5 ml) or so boiling water. Let the herb absorb the water for a few minutes. Apply a dab of the herb to the inside of your upper arm or wrist and cover with an adhesive strip. Leave in place 12 to 24 hours. If no irritation develops, the herb is generally safe to use.

ETHICAL WILDCRAFTING

Ethical wildcrafting, simply put, is the act of harvesting your herbs fresh from the wild and taking care that you don't overharvest the area. This means that after harvesting there is enough healthy, growing herb remaining on site to continue to spread and repopulate the surrounding environment.

United Plant Savers (see resources) is an organization that is dedicated to replanting endangered and threatened medicinal plants. Here is an excerpt from their brochure regarding wildcrafting.

◆ Always wildcraft with thoughts of beauty. Put beauty into your work. Ask yourself, "How much more beautiful will this plant community be when I am finished gathering?"

◆ Think first about the plant community and how many plants it can manage without, not how many plants you need in order to make products or profits.

◆ Treat the native plant complexes like the fine perennial gardens that they are.

◆ Do not upset in any manner undisturbed native soil — it is rare and precious.

◆ Take only as many plants as you can reasonably use; strive for zero waste.

◆ Replant the areas you are harvesting from. Scatter seeds, replace crowns and plant roots. Leave plenty of mature and seed-producing plants to reproduce.

◆ Start a replanting project in your area to help reestablish endangered and threatened species.

◆ Know the endangered plant species in your bio-region.

CLAY, SALT, THICKENERS, AND MISCELLANEOUS INGREDIENTS

This section outlines what I call "active ingredients," because they act as emulsifiers and binders, thickeners, humectants, preservatives, and pH balancers. These ingredients can be purchased through better health food and grocery stores, herb shops, and mail-order suppliers (see resources).

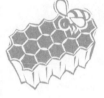

BEESWAX
Form Used: Pure, unrefined, filtered or unfiltered beeswax
Cosmetic Properties and Uses: A thickener for making lip balms, salves, creams, and lotions. Purchase fresh from an apiary, if possible.

BORAX
Form Used: Crystalline powdered mineral salt
Cosmetic Properties and Uses: Can be bought in the laundry aisle of grocery stores. Acts as a binder and texturizer and, when combined with beeswax, oil, and water, makes a stable emulsion. Also acts as a whitener, mild antiseptic, and natural preservative.

CLAY, FRENCH GREEN
Form Used: Dried powder
Cosmetic Properties and Uses: A sage-green, highly mineralized clay, it's especially good for oily skin and for healing conditions that need drawing, astringency, sloughing, or circulation stimulation, such as acne, eczema, psoriasis, and devitalized, wrinkled skin.

CLAY, WHITE COSMETIC
Form Used: Dried powder
Cosmetic Properties and Uses: Preferred in facial care products for sensitive or normal-to-dry skin because of its gentleness. I use it when making masks and scrubs. Draws impurities from your skin, exfoliates, and remineralizes your complexion.

COCOA BUTTER
Form Used: Fatty cocoa wax or butter
Cosmetic Properties and Uses: Acts as a soothing emollient to sunburned and dry skin. Use in lip balms, creams, and lotions to soften the skin and thicken the product. Hardens in cold weather, but melts when applied to the skin.

GLYCERIN, VEGETABLE
Form Used: Clear, sweet thick liquid
Cosmetic Properties and Uses: Acts as a humectant, which means it draws moisture from the air to your skin. Use in lotions and creams for dry skin. Makes lip balms taste super sweet!

GRAPEFRUIT SEED EXTRACT
Common Names: Grapefruit extract, citrus seed extract, citrus extract
Form Used: Concentrated liquid extract
Cosmetic Properties and Uses: Used mainly as an astringent preservative and antimicrobial in the cosmetic industry. I add it to facial and body splashes, creams, and lotions to extend the shelf life of the product.

LANOLIN, ANHYDROUS
Form Used: Fat or wax from sheep's wool
Cosmetic Properties and Uses: An emollient that holds water on the skin. It absorbs water and is a terrific emulsifier for creams and lotions.
Contraindication: May be a potential allergen — do a patch test first (as described on page 62).

SEA SALT
Form Used: Granular sea salt
Cosmetic Properties and Uses: Rich in minerals. Aids in healing oozing, itchy, rashy, inflamed skin. When added to bath water, sea salt can benefit skin afflicted with acne, eczema, psoriasis, poison plant rash, and other irritations.
Contraindication: Limit salt baths to 2 to 3 times per week as this mineral can be drying to the skin. Always follow a salt bath with an application of a good moisturizer.

WATER, DISTILLED
Form Used: Steam-distilled water
Cosmetic Properties and Uses: Used in making all cosmetic products that call for water or herb infusions. Will discourage premature mold growth in your cosmetics, which may occur if you use plain tap water.

WITCH HAZEL
Form Used: Liquid, water- and alcohol-based extract of witch hazel herb
Cosmetic Properties and Uses: Mild astringent. The ideal cleanser for minor cuts, scratches, and pimples. I use it as a facial splash base for normal-to-oily skin. The drugstore variety is fine.

WHAT DOES pH MEAN?

The pH (potential hydrogen) of a liquid refers to its degree of acidity or alkalinity. The pH scale goes from 0 to 14, with the neutral point being 7. Anything below a 7 on the pH scale is regarded as acid, and anything above 7 is considered alkaline. The lower the pH, the greater the degree of acidity; the higher the pH, the greater the degree of alkalinity. The pH of normal, healthy skin ranges from 4.5 to 6 and is most often given as 5.5.

Most soaps and shampoos have a pH value between 8 and 11, quite alkaline, while most toners and facial splashes have a pH value of between 4.5 and 6, more on the "skin-loving" acid side.

Your skin maintains its proper pH level by forming an acid mantle on its surface with the combined secretions of your sweat and oil glands. Using a toner after cleansing will keep your skin at its proper pH level, helping to prevent bacterial penetration (which can occur when skin is too acidic) and flaking and scaling due to moisture loss (which can occur when skin is too alkaline). Diluted herbal vinegars are ideal for restoring normal skin pH.

VINEGAR, RAW APPLE CIDER

Form Used: Diluted vinegar

Cosmetic Properties and Uses: Softens and relieves itchy skin if added to bath water. I use it as a base for making herbal splashes and toners for all skin types. The natural fruit acids in vinegar act as a gentle exfoliant, leaving skin smooth and glowing. Restores normal pH to skin after cleansing.

Contraindication: May irritate sensitive or sunburned skin.

VITAMIN E (D-ALPHA TOCOPHEROL)

Form Used: Liquid capsule form

Cosmetic Properties and Uses: Acts as a natural preservative and antioxidant when added to creams, lotions, and base oils. Helps prevent rancidity. Reported to soften and gradually fade scar tissue. Fabulous relief for chapped lips and ragged cuticles.

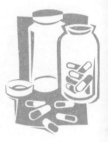

TOOLS, CONTAINERS, AND SUPPLIES

Whether preparing skin care products or dinner for six, the same sanitary precautions apply. Always wash your hands, pots, pans, knives, spoons, whisks, spatulas, blender, cutting board, and every other tool you'll be using in very hot, soapy water. You want to minimize the potential for harmful bacterial growth.

Containers for your final products should be sterilized. There are a few different methods you can use:

- ◆ Run them through the dishwasher.
- ◆ Soak them in very hot, soapy water combined with a bit of bleach (approximately 1 tablespoon (15 ml) for every gallon (4 l) of water) for approximately 15 minutes; then give them a good scrub to wash off the bleach.
- ◆ If you have glass containers, immerse them in boiling water for 1 minute.

Equipment

Preparing skin care products requires only common, everyday kitchen equipment. Here's a list of what you will need:

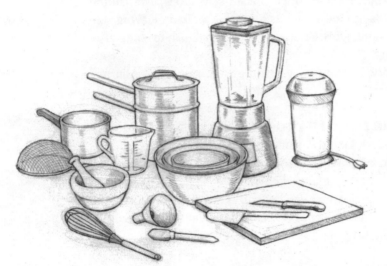

Most of the equipment and utensils you'll need for making your own herbal preparations can already be found right in your kitchen.

BLENDER

Blenders are useful for making lotions or creams in quantities of 1 cup or more. A blender can also be used to grind oatmeal, nuts, seeds, and herbs, but a nut/seed or coffee grinder does a much better job.

BOWLS

Use glass, plastic, stainless steel, enamel, or ceramic bowls. Make sure they're easy to clean and comfortable to hold. You'll need a variety of sizes, from the smallest ramekin for mixing single-serving facial scrubs to a large mixing bowl for facial steams.

COFFEE GRINDER

This kitchen gadget gets more use than any other piece of equipment I own. It's basically the same as a nut/seed grinder. I grind oatmeal, almonds, seeds, and flowers into powders for facial and body scrubs and masks. I use separate grinders for my cosmetics and my coffee — coffee beans leave a lingering flavor and aroma in the grinder that will permeate your natural skin care ingredients, tainting your products.

CUTTING BOARD

Used for slicing and dicing miscellaneous items. I keep a separate cutting board for processing any meat products. Always keep your boards extremely clean by washing them in hot, soapy water with a bit of bleach added for extra disinfecting.

DOUBLE BOILER

This piece of equipment is used to melt wax, cocoa butter, or coconut oil, and to warm oils when making various creams, lotions, and lip balms. The advantage of a double boiler is that it produces a gentle, even heat, making it impossible to scorch your ingredients if you suddenly get called away from the kitchen. If you don't have a double boiler, a basic stainless steel pan (or pans) to melt and warm ingredients is fine if placed over the lowest setting on the stove and its contents stirred occasionally.

EYEDROPPERS

Glass eyedroppers are useful for measuring essential oils by the drop. I try to have a separate one for each oil. Sterilize your droppers every so often by pouring rubbing alcohol through them. Purchase droppers from mail-order herb supply stores, craft stores, bottle companies, or drugstores.

FUNNELS

A small funnel (plastic or stainless steel) comes in handy when pouring liquid recipes into narrow-necked storage bottles. Funnels come in various sizes and are available in most hardware and grocery stores.

MEASURING CUPS AND SPOONS

Preparing creams and lotions frequently requires exacting measurements; that's where these come in handy.

MORTAR AND PESTLE

Usually available in three sizes, approximately 3, 4½, or 6 inches (7.5, 11.3, or 15 cm) in diameter, and made from marble, polished granite, colored and sandblasted glass, or wood. I prefer the larger stone variety because of its heft. Perfect for crushing dried seeds, herbs, and spices; for mashing fresh herbs, flowers, and blackberries or raspberries to extract their juices; and to make spreadable pulp pastes from fruits such as pineapple, papaya, and strawberries. These are sold in better hardware stores, kitchen supply stores, some herb shops and health food stores, or through mail-order suppliers.

POTS AND PANS

Stainless steel, enamel, or glass only, please. Best to have a variety of sizes, including a 1-pint (500 ml) saucepan and 1-, 2-, and 3-quart (1-, 2-, and 3-liter) pots. I use all sizes for melting oils and beeswax as well as for making herb tea and extracting mucilaginous substances from herb roots.

CHOOSING POTS AND PANS

Fruits, herbal teas, and herbal vinegars contain acids, tannins, and resins that may react with aluminum, cast iron, teflon, or copper. To avoid product discoloration or other adverse reactions in your skin care formulas, use only stainless steel, glass, or enamel pans.

PARING KNIVES

I always have several sharp blades at my disposal. I cut beeswax with a paring knife instead of using a cheese grater. It's easier on my knuckles! Be sure to keep your knives sharp. My good friend Hervé works as a produce clerk at the local grocery store and is constantly opening boxes and crates using a big, sharp knife. He informs me that most knife injuries are the result of using a dull knife, not a sharp one. "A dull knife," he says, "requires more pressure on your part to cut a piece of fruit, an herb stem, or a vegetable, thus increasing the likelihood of slipping and cutting your finger instead."

SPATULA

A spatula is better than a spoon for scooping out creams and lotions from any type of container. I recommend keeping a variety of sizes on hand.

STRAINER

I use a woven bamboo or standard mesh strainer for straining liquids that contain large herb matter. For straining finely ground materials, I line either of these strainers with cheesecloth or a nylon stocking.

WHISK

A small wire whisk is great for blending and whipping a small quantity of lotion, cream, salve, or lip balm.

Containers

Obviously, if you make an herbal product you have to store it in something, and the more attractive the container, the better. Cosmetic companies know that packaging sells — frequently the pretty package costs more to produce than the ingredients inside! What I'm trying to say is this: If you store your fresh rosemary face cream in an old mustard jar, you won't be as apt to use it as you would if you stored it in an aesthetically pleasing jar.

Discount import/export shops and flea markets often carry scads of bottles and jars for the herbal crafter at really great prices. Herb shops and health food stores, though, can be rather expensive places to purchase individual bottles. Antiques shops often sell really unique containers if you're looking for something special. I generally purchase my containers by the case from mail-order bottle companies (see resources). As always, buying in bulk saves money.

Don't forget to label your skin care creations. A simple custom label looks professional and your friends will want to purchase some of your wares for gift-giving. Ever thought of starting an herbal craft business? If so, check out the following informative books: *Growing Your Herb Business* and *Creating an Herbal Bodycare Business* (see Suggested Reading).

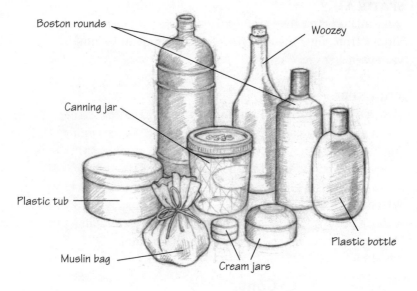

Boston rounds

Woozey

Canning jar

Plastic tub

Muslin bag

Cream jars

Plastic bottle

There are a multitude of containers to choose from for storing your preparations and formulas, including but not limited to the ones shown here.

BOSTON ROUNDS

A Boston round is a glass container perfect for spritzers, lotions, and oils. They come in myriad colors: amber, clear, green, and cobalt blue, and in sizes from ½ ounce to 16 ounces (15 to 450 g). Darker colored glass will protect your herbal products from light damage. They can be topped with a simple plastic cap, lotion pump, glass dropper, or mister.

CANNING JARS

From half-pint to gallon (250 ml to 4 liter) size, these are suitable for storing dried herbs. The half-pint size is perfect for packaging your wares to give to friends. Slap on your custom label and *voilà!* you've got a beautiful present!

CREAM JARS

Available in different sizes from ¼- to 4-ounce (7- to 115-g) jars. Perfect for creams, lip balms, and healing salves. Available in glass or plastic.

MUSLIN BAGS

Available in a variety of sizes and are useful for making bath bags or large quantities of herbal tea. They are easy to make or can be purchased from craft stores or mail-order suppliers.

PLASTIC BOTTLES

From 2 ounces to 16 ounces (60 to 500 ml), and larger. These can be used for the same products as Boston rounds, except they do not protect the herbal contents from light damage. Better to use if you travel or frequently have children in your bathroom.

PLASTIC TUBS

These are plastic food storage containers with a good-fitting, airtight lid, available in all grocery stores. I use them to store dry facial and body scrubs and mask blends.

WOOZEYS

Designed mainly for culinary use as wine and vinegar bottles, these narrow-necked bottles are super for storing facial and body splashes, floral waters, and bath oils.

FOR SAFETY'S SAKE

Though most of the ingredients in the skin care recipes included in this book are safe to consume, some, essential oils for example, can be quite harmful. Please label each product you make and store away from pets and children.

CHAPTER 6
Natural Solutions for
Common Skin Problems

▼▼▼

It's time to face your complexion challenges armed with knowledge. Because your skin is a living, complex system of intertwining processes, your focus needs to shift from merely addressing symptoms to actually supporting the healthy functioning of your skin. Attune your skin. Let it reflect a harmonious balance between the internal workings of your body and the exposure it receives from its external environment.

Whether your quest is to postpone the inevitability of aging, cure your cystic acne, lighten your age spots, educate yourself about skin cancer prevention, or quench your dry skin's thirst, you've come to the right spot. Dermatological medications and topical chemical treatments are occasionally necessary to help manage troublesome skin afflictions, but these drugs can have irritating and even potentially irreversible side effects and should be avoided whenever possible. I feel that 90 percent of the time there is a natural solution to every health problem that crosses your path. Common skin maladies are not an exception.

Remember, achieving flawless skin is not an instantaneous process. Nature takes time to work her magic. Your skin didn't assume its present condition overnight, so have patience. In time, your skin will reveal the true beauty within you.

A good, holistically oriented dermatologist can help guide you through the maze of toxic treatments and design a beneficial treatment plan you can live with. An esthetician trained in holistic skin care can be of assistance in designing a skin care program to augment your dermatologist's recommendations and can also show you how to properly care for your skin at home.

The advice of your dermatologist and esthetician can prove invaluable when it comes to matters of the skin, but

A **dermatologist** is a medical doctor specializing in disorders of the skin. A dermatologist can prescribe drugs and perform surgical procedures.

An **esthetician** is someone who has completed a specified amount of training in esthetics required by his or her state (usually between 300 to 600 hours). An esthetician usually has training in specialties such as makeup artistry, aromatherapy, nutrition, massage, reflexology, manual lymph drainage, waxing, and pre- and postoperative skin care.

remember — only you can take control of your appearance and health. The more you strive to live in harmony with your surroundings, eat a nutritious diet, and take proper care of your skin, the more benefits your skin will reap. So, read on and take charge of your skin's health. Only you can change the outlook of the skin you're in!

ACNE

Acne vulgaris, or acne, as it is commonly known, is the most common skin disease. Acneic skin is oily, shiny, and blemished and has enlarged pores (which are often clogged) and blackheads and whiteheads covering its surface. Acne manifests on the face and frequently on the neck, chest, shoulders, and back. Pimples can be red and inflamed and, if not properly addressed, can lead to larger pimples (pustules) and deeper lumps (cysts or nodules). More often than not, a person who suffers from acne will have oily hair as well, which exacerbates the problem by causing breakouts around the hairline.

Causes of Acne

According to dermatologists, acne is caused by the hormone testosterone, which stimulates production of oil (sebum),

According to the American Academy of Dermatology, more than 80 percent of the country's teenagers will suffer from some degree of acne.

which promotes acne. It is not caused by poor hygiene, but it can be aggravated by improper skin care, high heat and humidity, stress, and improper diet.

Acne begins when a sebaceous follicle is obstructed by a combination of cellular debris and sebum. This obstruction forms a *comedone*, or plug, commonly referred to as either a blackhead (if it has a brown or black head) or a whitehead or milia (if it has a white head). If a whitehead ruptures beneath the surface of the skin, either involuntarily or because it was squeezed or improperly extracted, a chain reaction is triggered. First a pimple forms, which becomes inflamed as bacteria begin to grow in the surrounding tissue. Now this simple pimple has become a pustule and looks red and angry, filled with yellow pus. If the situation worsens and the infection moves deeper, a painful, inflamed nodule could form, which looks like an ugly, round knot on the skin. Should the nodule progress, a sac filled with fluid forms, called a cyst. Cysts are deep, serious lesions that require medical treatment.

There are four grades of acne:

Grade I: In mild cases of acne vulgaris, the skin displays a few minor pimples, whiteheads, and blackheads.

Grade II: The skin has more pimples and/or pustules (a pimple containing pus), and pores are more frequently clogged.

Grade III: The skin displays a greater inflammation of lesions in the form of pustules (large and small) and a further increase in blackhead and whitehead development.

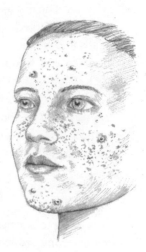

In the Grade II level of acne, whiteheads, blackheads, and pustules are obvious.

Grade IV: Many large pustules, nodules (deep pustules), and cysts are often accompanied by areas heavily congested with blackheads and whiteheads. This grade of acne should be treated only by a dermatologist.

Acne is not just for adolescents. True, acne commonly rears its ugly head with the hormonal surge of the preteen years, but many cases occur in adults, especially women. Adult-onset acne tends to be due to increased stress, overzealous cleansing, and the hormonal changes of pregnancy, menstrual cycles, menopause, or as a result of hormonal abnormalities, including the increased testosterone productivity that may accompany ovarian cysts. Unlike teenage acne, adult acne usually confines itself to the chin and jawline areas, though I've also seen it flare up on the nose and cheeks.

Although both men and women respond to stress with a rise in adrenal hormones, women, in particular, respond by overproducing testosterone, thereby causing adult-onset acne. Just how does increased stress induce acne? According to Robert and Webster Stone, authors of *Zit Wars: The Battle for Great Skin,* stress activates the hypothalamus, which stimulates the pituitary gland, thus stimulating the adrenal glands, which then release testosterone, stimulating the oil glands to produce oil (sebum), which promotes acne.

HANDS OFF!

Remember as a teen when your mother told you not to pick at your blemishes because it could make them worse? Well, she was right! Self-treatment of acne, including picking or squeezing with fingernails, needles, or metal implements is not helpful. It can cause your simple pimple to rupture under the surface of the skin, become inflamed, and lead to either a permanent pitted scar or possibly an ugly, painful cyst. There is a correct way to "pop" your pimples — see page 87.

Prevention

Here is a bit of sage advice toward the prevention of this annoying skin disease:

Identify your skin type. Take care of your skin, treat it well, and it will bless you with years of beauty. Neglect it, and it can be the bane of your existence. See a skin professional and find out what type of skin you have and how to properly take care of its needs, then follow their recommendations to the letter.

Choose cosmetics wisely. Ideally, facial makeup, lotions, and creams should be hypoallergenic, noncomedogenic, and nonacnegenic; these products are unlikely to cause allergies and and won't clog your pores. *Acne cosmetica* is the term for cosmetic-induced acne and is quite common.

Supplement your diet. Some supplements, such as vitamin A, zinc, cod liver oil, borage oil, and evening primrose oil, have been shown to be helpful in many cases of acne, from mild to severe (see chapter 2 for more information). Cod liver oil and evening primrose oil have indeed been a blessing to my mild case of adult-onset acne. I take one tablespoon of cod liver oil every other day and one 1,300 mg capsule of evening primrose oil daily.

Be gentle to your skin. Avoid overzealous cleansing of your skin as well as industrial strength facial scrubs. In an attempt to rid themselves of pimples and blackheads — which, incidentally, can't be washed away — many sufferers scrub their faces with either a washcloth and soap or an exfoliant product, several times a day, like it was the kitchen floor. This acts only to dry the skin's surface and stimulate more oil production beneath. Use a gentle hand and soothing, mild products specifically designed for your skin type when cleansing.

Practice stress reduction. I can't emphasize this enough! If you're an adult woman suffering with adult-onset acne, I can almost guarantee that your disturbing skin condition will subside if you lower the stress in your life. Yoga, reiki, reflexology, walking, running, rollerblading, meditation, gardening . . . whatever it takes for you to relax, partake of it frequently. The less stress in your life, the less adrenaline and testosterone your body will produce.

Beware of iodine intake. A few sensitive individuals experience irritation of the follicles when excess iodides in the diet are excreted through the sebaceous ducts. To determine if iodine is aggravating your acne, minimize or avoid foods containing iodides, such as kelp, liver, fish and shellfish, corn, white onions, asparagus, milk, and beef. Certain supplements contain high levels of iodine too, so check the label. Additionally, some brands of birth control pills contain iodides — ask your doctor if your brand contains iodides, and if so, ask for a different prescription.

Hydrate. Drink plenty of pure water to flush out toxins and keep the skin hydrated.

Sleep well. If you "party hearty" too often, it will show up on your skin. Eight hours of sleep each night (or whatever it takes to make you feel rested and lively) is imperative.

Avoid stimulants. Stay away from or limit stimulants such as caffeine and cigarettes. They sap valuable nutrients that are essential for skin health, such as vitamins B and C, from your system.

Don't touch. Keep your hands off your face. If you have oily hair, shampoo daily and keep your hair in a style that is up and off your face.

Treatments for Acne

To heal or at least lessen the severity of your acne, you must normalize or attempt to reduce the sebum production in your skin. This can be accomplished in several ways. Drug therapy could include topical treatments such as benzoyl peroxide; salicylic-acid lotions, creams, and toners; tretinoin; sodium sulfacetamide lotion; or Retin-A. Accutane, an oral medication, is very popular and extremely effective, but can have terrible side effects and its use must be monitored by a dermatologist. If your acne is severe, other oral antibiotics such as tetracycline, minocycline, or erythromycin might be prescribed. Though these therapies can be successful by reducing bacteria and comedone formation, they can have unfortunate side effects that range from facial and oral dryness and chapped lips to birth defects in pregnant women.

Alternatively, you could choose a more natural, holistically supportive approach to treating your complexion, *sans* side effects. There are many gentle yet effective herbal tonics and natural cleansers that can be used to encourage more harmonious functioning of your skin.

Regardless of which route you choose, your acne will not heal overnight. Dermatologists say to allow at least 1 to 6 months for your problem skin to show signs of improvement. In order to head off future acne eruptions, you must adhere to a strict regimen of home and professional care. Make a commitment to stick with your treatments. Consistency is the key to clearer skin.

FACE IT

This herbal tea, formulated by Jean Argus of Jean's Greens, is a tasty way to nourish your body and aid in liver detoxification. It comes from an old Mexican formula and is used daily to improve skin. It's available in bulk from her mail-order catalog. I highly recommend it.

    4 tablespoons (60 ml) dried oatstraw
    4 tablespoons (60 ml) dried figwort
    2 tablespoons (30 ml) dried sarsaparilla
    2 tablespoons (30 ml) dried burdock
    1½ teaspoons (7.5 ml) dried yellow dock
    ½ teaspoon (2.5 ml) dried licorice root
    1 teaspoon (5 ml) dried stevia (to sweeten)

To make: To 4 cups (1 liter) of boiling water, add 4–6 heaping teaspoons (20–30 ml) of tea and immediately remove from heat. Cover and steep for 10–15 minutes. Strain and cool if desired.

To use: Consume 4 cups (1 liter) daily as an internal skin tonic. For maximum benefit, continue regular consumption over 4–6 months to see desired results.

Yield: Enough for approximately 30–35 cups (7.5–9 l) of tea

Liver tonics. The liver is primarily responsible for keeping hormones such as testosterone in check. Most herbalists, if asked to recommend a formula for clearing the skin of chronic skin problems such as eczema, psoriasis, rashes, or acne, will usually include herbs to improve the functioning of the liver, such as those in the Face It tea formula (see page 80).

Natural cleansers. Acneic skin should be kept scrupulously clean and the follicles regularly deep cleansed and kept that way to prevent future breakouts. The cleansing products you choose should be water-based and free of perfumes, dyes, and most chemicals. Your aim is to thoroughly clean but not strip your skin's protective acid barrier. Always rinse with tepid (not hot) water, followed by an herbal toner (such as my Yarrow Skin Toner) and an oil-free moisturizer or aromatic hydrosol spray to prevent dehydration.

YARROW SKIN TONER

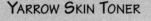

This astringent liquid will serve as an effective herbal antiseptic to kill the bacteria that accompanies acne development, help balance the production of excess sebum, and reduce the visible oil on your face. I recommend it for normal, oily, or acneic complexions.

2 cups (500 ml) boiling water
2 heaping teaspoons (10 ml) dried yarrow or 4 heaping teaspoons (20 ml) fresh
10 drops tea tree essential oil
5 drops inula graveolens or eucalyptus essential oil

To make: Add yarrow to boiling water, remove from heat, cover and steep for 30 minutes until nice and strong. Strain and cool. Add essential oils. Store in a jar or squeeze bottle in the refrigerator for up to 1 month.
To use: May be applied using a cotton square as a toner to your entire face or body after cleansing, or whenever you need degreasing. Feels especially good if chilled and splashed on post-workouts.
Yield: 2 cups (500 ml)

Regular exfoliation through the use of alpha- or beta-hydroxy acid products or clay-based masks is of utmost importance to help reduce breakouts and remove dead skin buildup that could clog pores. Use one of my gentle exfoliation recipes (such as the Anti-Aging Formula on page 180) or find a mild natural product that includes soothing ingredients such as German chamomile, lavender, comfrey, and calendula.

Sebum maintenance. I live in a coastal community on Cape Cod, Massachusetts, and when the summer heat and humidity strike in July and August, my normal-to-dry skin does an about-face and pumps out the oil. For 2 months I alter my cleansing routine to remove the excess oil and shine. I rely on gentle soaps from my natural products company, September's Sun Herbal Soap & Skin Care, that are very gentle and don't strip my skin of all its protective oils. After a cleansing with natural soap, I apply an herbal toner and follow up with the Sebum Balancing Formula, which helps to reduce and balance the oil production in my skin.

SEBUM BALANCING FORMULA

2 tablespoons (30 ml) almond or hazelnut oil
4 drops spike lavender essential oil
4 drops eucalyptus essential oil
3 drops blue cypress essential oil
2 drops lemongrass essential oil (optional)

To make: Combine all ingredients in a small, 1-ounce (30-ml) glass bottle, and cap tightly. Store formula in a refrigerator for up to 1 year.

To use: Apply on clean, damp skin after using an aromatic hydrosol or toner. Place 2–4 drops in the palm of your hand and add a few drops of water. Rub palms together to warm and mix the liquids and then press gently onto your face and neck. Don't rub or massage your face too aggressively. Your skin should rapidly absorb this formula.

Yield: 1 ounce (30 ml)

Treating Blackhead Outbreaks

Blackheads can develop singularly or in clusters anywhere the skin is particularly oily, especially the face, neck, shoulders, chest, and back. At times they appear flush with the skin's surface and are barely detectable and other times are slightly raised, very black, and obvious. If infected, a blackhead may be surrounded by pus.

Blackheads are formed by obstructions in your pores, or hair follicles. Oil-producing sebaceous glands, which are connected to your hair follicles, secrete a mixture of fats, proteins, cholesterol, and inorganic salts onto the surface of your skin to keep it supple, hold in moisture, and keep your hair pliable and shiny. When your pores (follicles) become filled with solidified sebum, bacteria, and keratinized skin cells, the oil plug moves upward and outward, dilating the opening of the pore and making it quite visible. The blackness is not caused by dirt; rather, a combination of skin pigment cells and exposure to oxygen gives the oil plug its color. A whitehead, on the other hand, has a layer of skin covering it and has not been exposed to oxygen; it remains white.

To prevent the formation of these unsightly black oil plugs and enlarged pores, your skin must be kept deep-down clean. Cleanse twice daily with an oil-free cleanser, then apply an herbal toner for oily skin (such as strong peppermint or sage tea) or an aromatic hydrosol. Follow up with an oil-free moisturizer if necessary. An oil-absorbing clay mask, such as the Fruit Paste Mask (see page 84), should be used in blackhead prone areas once or twice a week to absorb excess oil and exfoliate dead skin cells.

QUICK BLACKHEAD CLEANSER

To prevent blackheads, try this quick formula for a cleanser: 1 teaspoon (5 ml) liquid castile soap (available in most health food stores) mixed with 1 drop tea tree or thyme essential oil. You can mix it right at the sink as you're washing up.

Fruit Paste Mask

A simple yet effective treatment for blackhead outbreaks.

1 tablespoon (15 ml) white cosmetic clay
2 teaspoons (10 ml) freshly squeezed apple, pineapple, or grape juice

To make: Combine ingredients in a small bowl and stir until a smooth, spreadable paste forms. If the paste is too thick, add more juice; if too runny, add a bit more clay.

To use: Spread a thick paste over freshly cleansed, blackhead prone area(s) and allow to dry completely, approximately 20 minutes. Rinse with cool or tepid water. Pat dry and apply a dab of oil-free moisturizer mixed with a drop of tea tree or eucalyptus essential oil to the area. May be used once or twice weekly or as needed to keep pores clean and clear.

Yield: 1 treatment

Blackhead Extraction Procedure

Blackheads can be removed by extraction. When the oil plug is removed the pore will appear smaller, but since the pore has been enlarged and filled with a blackhead, chances are it will become filled again in a few weeks unless you are extra diligent about your skin care regimen.

You'll need:

◆ Two squares of flannel cloth, large enough to comfortably wrap around your index fingers
◆ A washcloth
◆ A bowl holding 4 to 5 cups (1,000 to 1,250 ml) of very warm water or chamomile tea
◆ Two tablespoons (30 ml) Epsom salts or sea salt

Step 1: Cleanse the skin thoroughly with a gentle, oil-free cleanser.

Step 2: Stir the salt into the warm water or tea and stir until dissolved.

Step 3: Soak the washcloth in the salty water and squeeze out the excess liquid. Place washcloth over blackhead(s) you wish to extract and hold it there for about 5 minutes to soften the skin and sebum and ready the skin for extraction. Concentrate on one area of your face or body at a time.

Step 4: When ready, dampen the flannel squares in the same liquid as you did the washcloth and then wrap them around your index fingers. While holding the skin taut between your two fingers, begin a very gentle squeezing and lifting motion on either side of the blackhead. Do not apply too much pressure. You should see a semi-solid white or yellow waxy secretion exude from the pore opening. If you don't, then the blackhead is not ready to come out and if you proceed, you'll only damage the surrounding tissue and possibly cause a nasty pimple. Continue this procedure on other blackheads.

Step 5: Following the extraction, use the Fruit Paste Mask (see page 84) on the treated areas to remove even more sebum, minimize pore size, and reduce possible inflammation. Add a drop of German chamomile or everlasting essential oil to the recipe, as these ingredients have powerful anti-inflammatory properties.

Treating Pimple Outbreaks

Everyone is well aware of what a pesky pimple looks like. That red, slightly raised spot that may or may not be infected with a creamy yellow center (pus) seems to always appear at just the wrong time and in the wrong place. I'm not discussing full-fledged acne here, just a minor pimple outbreak and how to deal with it.

When a pore or hair follicle becomes clogged by excess dead skin cells, sebum, and bacteria and ruptures beneath the skin, a pimple forms. A breakout can be triggered by stress, hormone fluctuation, improper cleansing, and overactive sebaceous glands. You don't have to have particularly oily skin to have a pimple, or two or three. I sometimes break out during the winter when my skin tends to be dehydrated. Everyone gets a pimple from time to time; no one is completely immune.

Quick tips. Here are some valuable points to consider to help prevent the occasional pimple. You may recognize some of the advice, as it was given earlier for treating acne, and indeed you'll find the same advice repeated throughout this chapter. The point? Even if you have relatively healthy, problem-free skin, you still need to follow good skin care basics in order to maintain a vibrant complexion.

- Keep your hands off your face.
- Stick to a proper cleansing regimen for your skin type.
- If you spend lots of time on the telephone, sanitize it daily and apply an astringent toner to your lower cheek, jawline, and neck.
- Avoid restrictive clothing if possible, or at least apply a bit of medicated cornstarch or arrowroot powder to absorb perspiration and keep the area dry and relatively friction-free.
- Grow out your bangs and get them off your face, or keep your hair scrupulously clean and oil free.
- Get rid of the stress in your life or at least minimize it.
- Get plenty of exercise and fresh air, and eat a healthy diet.
- Drink plenty of water to flush toxins from your system and keep your skin hydrated.

Tea tree oil. According to an article in the August 1998 issue of *Vegetarian Times* by Norine Dworkin, "Tea tree oil is known as an effective acne fighter. A 1990 study by Lederle Laboratories and Royal Prince Alfred Hospital in Great Britain found that a 5 percent tea tree oil gel was as effective as benzoyl peroxide in treating acne, with less drying, stinging, and redness. Use a commercially prepared ointment, available in natural health stores, or dab undiluted oil right on pimples."

Yes, tea tree essential oil is a wonderful spot treatment. Its antiseptic and antibacterial properties make it a superior choice for fighting pimples whenever they arise.

PIMPLE MAGIC JUICE

This essential oil formula really seems to help heal breakouts in a hurry!

> 2 tablespoons (30 ml) store-bought aloe vera juice
> 2 drops thyme essential oil (chemotype linalol)
> 2 drops tea tree essential oil
> 2 drops spike lavender essential oil
> 2 drops eucalyptus essential oil

To make: Combine all ingredients in a 1-ounce (30-ml) bottle and shake well. Store in a cool, dry, dark place for up to 4 months, or refrigerate for up to 1 year.
To use: Dab directly on pimple after cleansing. May use up to 3 times daily. If irritation occurs, reduce usage.
Yield: 1 ounce

PIMPLE EXTRACTION PROCEDURE

To effectively "pop" a pimple, the pimple must first come to a very visible head with the pus showing prominently in the center. A layer of crust may have formed over the top. Do not attempt to extract any pimples that do not have this appearance or you could cause scarring or the formation of a cyst.

You'll need:

- ◆ Two squares of flannel cloth, large enough to comfortably wrap around your index fingers
- ◆ A washcloth
- ◆ A sewing needle
- ◆ A bowl holding 4 to 5 cups (1,000 to 1,250 ml) of very warm water or pepperment tea
- ◆ 4 drops thyme essential oil
- ◆ 2 drops German chamomile essential oil
- ◆ 2 tablespoons (30 ml) Epsom salts or sea salt
- ◆ Matches or rubbing alcohol

Step 1: Cleanse the area thoroughly.

Step 2: Add the essential oils and salt to the warm water or tea. Stir until the salt is dissolved.

Step 3: Soak the washcloth in the salty water and squeeze out the excess liquid. Hold the cloth over the pimple for a few minutes to soften the sebum, which will make extraction easier.

Step 4: Sterilize a needle in a match flame or rubbing alcohol. Use it to prick the center surface skin of the pimple carefully, to open the top layer of epidermis. This ensures that the pus will break through on the surface of the skin and not be pushed into the lower layers, where it could cause further inflammation.

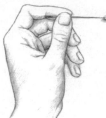

Be careful to prick just the top layer of skin over the pimple.

Step 5: When ready, dampen the flannel squares in the same liquid as you did the washcloth and then wrap them around your index fingers. (*Do not* use your fingernails, as they can cause scars.) Apply gentle pressure on each side of the pimple with a lifting, slightly squeezing motion. The debris should ooze from the clogged pore. If it doesn't, try twice more on different sides of the pimple, then stop. You don't want to cause deeper damage. Blood or clear fluid should ooze from the pore following the pus extraction.

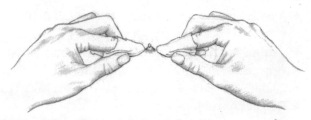

Gently apply a lifting, slightly squeezing pressure to force the debris up and out from the clogged pore.

Step 6: Apply Pimple Magic Juice (see page 87) or a dab of tea tree essential oil to the area to cleanse and disinfect.

Consulting the Experts

See an Esthetician If: An esthetician can be of great assistance in the care of acneic skin. She can provide a gentle facial or back treatment and steam or hot packs to soften the skin and loosen hardened sebum. Depending on the severity of your condition, she may suggest a series of deep-pore cleansings to thoroughly remove the pore-clogging debris, and will often work in conjunction with any prescribed dermatological treatments. Additionally, she can educate you as to which home treatment products are most beneficial for your particular skin condition.

See a Dermatologist If: Some skin conditions, such as severe cystic or nodular acne, require the care of a doctor. If your acne is unresponsive to home treatments and visits to an esthetician are not producing the desired results, consult a dermatologist. Locate a doctor who is holistically oriented, one who will treat your whole person — mind, body, and spirit — and not just the symptomatic spots on your face.

AGE SPOTS

See Hyperpigmentation on page 130.

CANCER

The incidence of skin cancer is rising at an alarming rate. My dermatologist, Dr. William W. Fiske of Yarmouthport, Massachusetts, told me that he sees approximately one new case of malignant melanoma per week — a significant increase from a decade ago. His advice to me was to avoid the sun completely if possible, to get my vitamin D requirement through diet or supplementation instead of the sun, and, if I must go outside, to wear a sunscreen with an SPF of at least 30. The sunscreen should provide UVA protection in addition to UVB protection, as the UVA rays cause the most skin damage.

THE COLD HARD FACTS

According to a March 1997 report from the American Academy of Dermatology, "Americans have a 1 in 84 risk for developing melanoma in their lifetime, an 1800% increase from 1930. One person each hour dies from malignant melanoma. Sixty-seven years ago, the lifetime risk for an American to develop an invasive melanoma was just one in 1,500. In 1980, the risk was one in 150. If the current rate of increase continues, it is estimated that by the year 2000, the lifetime risk will increase to one in 75. . . . Melanoma is the most frequent cancer in women ages 25–29 and the second most frequent in women ages 30–34, after breast cancer."

The Skin Cancer Foundation states that "the incidence of malignant melanoma is rising faster than almost any other cancer in the U.S. — doubling every ten years. One in five people afflicted with melanoma die of this cancer. Fortunately, melanoma is one of the easiest tumors to find and one of the easiest to cure, *if it is found and removed early.*"

Basal cell carcinoma was once primarily found in middle-aged or elderly patients but is now increasingly seen in the younger set, due to frequent, unprotected sun exposure. This cancer is rather slow growing and usually doesn't spread to other parts of the body. If left untreated, however, it can invade tissues beneath the skin, including bone.

Squamous cell carcinoma originates in the mid-to-upper levels of the epidermis and is commonly found on the sun-exposed areas of the body, such as the neck, head, ears, lips, and back of the hands. This cancer accounts for approximately 20 percent of all skin cancers. Squamous cell cancers are more aggressive than basal cell cancers and are more likely to invade tissues beneath the skin and to spread to more distant parts of the body.

Malignant melanoma is the least common but most deadly form of skin cancer, representing about 5 percent of all skin-related cancers. It originates just beneath or between the cells of the stratum basale (the base layer of the epidermis), where melanocytes (melanin-producing cells, or the cells that give your skin its color) are produced. Melanoma is characterized by the uncontrolled growth of melanocytes and can appear suddenly on any part of the body, but most frequently on the legs of women and on the upper back of women and men. If undetected in its early stages, melanoma can spread to other organs and may result in death.

SKINFORMATION

"As few as four visits a year to a tanning salon could quadruple your likelihood of getting melanoma," states Kathleen M. Carney in the June 1998 issue of *Smart Skin Care*. "Most beds block the UVB rays (the burning rays), but fail to block the UVA rays (the aging rays), which actually go deeper in the skin and cause more harm."

Causes of Skin Cancer

The comforting, warming, bright, cheery sun is the chief villain, I'm afraid. It's not that the sun is bad — it's necessary for all life on this beautiful planet of ours. It's the ultraviolet rays of the sun, or rather, the abuse or excessive exposure to ultraviolet radiation that can cause skin cancer.

Skin cancer can also result, though infrequently, from ionizing radiation (found in X rays), tanning beds, and exposure to particular chemicals. Studies are also being done to determine if mutant or abnormal genes can be inherited and increase a child's risk of developing skin cancer.

Are you at risk? Risk factors include fair skin, light eyes, freckles, skin that burns easily, red, blonde, or light-brown hair, the presence of many moles, family history of skin cancer, a suppressed immune system, and overexposure to ultraviolet radiation.

Identifying Skin Cancer

Skin cancer prevention organizations use the ABCD rule as a tool to help you tell a normal, harmless mole from one that might be a melanoma. Here it is:

A normal, benign mole will have even edges and a symmetrical shape. If divided down the middle, each half would be identical.

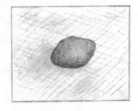

Normal

A for Asymmetry. Many forms of early melanoma are asymmetrical, which means that if divided down the middle, one half would not match the other.

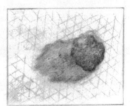

A for asymmetry

B for Border. Most early melanomas have borders that are uneven having ragged, notched, or scalloped edges.

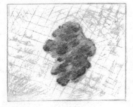

B for border

C for Color. Normal moles are often a single shade of light or dark brown or are flesh colored. Frequently, one of the first signs of a malignant melanoma is the appearance of varying shades of brown, tan, or black within a mole. If allowed to progress, blue, red, and white may also appear.

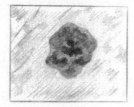

C for color

D for Diameter. The average benign mole is usually less than ¼ inch (6 mm) in diameter — about the size of a pencil eraser. Early melanomas tend to grow larger than a common mole. Any growth of a mole should alert you that something unusual is going on.

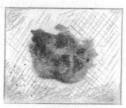

D for diameter

While the ABCD rule is a good guide to discovering a potential melanoma, there are always exceptions to the rule, so it's wise to take notice of any changes in skin lesions and bring them to the attention of your dermatologist.

Preventing Skin Cancer

Your chances of getting skin cancer can be greatly reduced if you follow these tips (from the American Academy of Dermatology):

- Try to avoid the sun between 10 A.M. and 4 P.M., when the sun's rays are the strongest.
- Apply a broad-spectrum sunscreen with a sun protection factor (SPF) of at least 15.
- Reapply sunscreen every 2 hours when outdoors, even on cloudy days.
- Wear protective, tightly woven clothing, such as a long-sleeved shirt and pants.
- Wear a 4-inch (10-cm) wide-brimmed hat and sunglasses, even when walking short distances.
- Stay in the shade whenever possible.
- Avoid reflective surfaces, which can reflect up to 85 percent of the sun's damaging rays.
- Protect children by keeping them out of the sun, minimizing sun exposure and applying sunscreens beginning at 6 months of age.
- If you notice a change in the size, shape, or appearance of a mole, see a dermatologist.

Treatments

Skin cancer is not treatable using a home remedy, but fortunately most skin cancers, including melanoma, can be cured if detected in the early stages of the disease. Most dermatologists recommend that you perform a monthly self-examination of your skin. Just as men should do a routine prostate self-examination and women a monthly breast self-examination, a monthly examination of your skin should be added to the list of body inspections.

To do this examination correctly, you'll need paper and pencil, a full-length mirror, a hand mirror, and a couple of chairs or ideally, a very close partner or friend. Just what exactly are you looking for? A new mole, existing mole, beauty mark, birthmark, freckle, or any growth or mark that has increased in size, shape, thickness, or is bigger than ¼ inch

(6 mm — the size of a pencil eraser), and appears tan, brown, black, translucent, pearly, or multicolored, such as white, red, blue, and black. A spot, lump, or sore that refuses to heal and continues to be painful, bleed, scab, or grow in size is also a sign that all is not right with your skin. This examination procedure is adapted from the Skin Cancer Foundation's brochure on self-examination, *Skin Cancer: If You Can Spot It, You Can Stop It.*

Step 1. Begin with your head. Examine your face, especially your nose, eyes, ears (front and back), lips, and mouth. You may need to use one mirror in front and one in the rear to get a good view.

Step 2. Thoroughly inspect your scalp, using a blow dryer and mirror to expose each section to view. I had a hard time doing this one by myself; a family member or friend comes in handy for this step.

Step 3. Check your hands and forearms. Look carefully between each finger and under your fingernails, where skin cancer can appear as a dark spot. Proceed up your forearms, checking front and back sides.

Step 4. Standing in front of a full-length mirror, beginning at the elbows, scan all sides of your upper arms, including your underarms.

Step 5. Now, focus on the front of the neck, chest, and torso. Women should lift each breast and examine underneath.

Step 6. With your back to a full-length mirror, use the hand mirror to inspect the back of your shoulders and neck, your upper back, and any part of your upper arms you could not view in Step 4.

Step 7. Still using both mirrors, take a look at your lower back, buttocks, between your buttocks and crotch area, and backs of both legs.

Step 8. Sitting down in a chair, prop each leg in turn on the other stool or chair. Using the hand mirror, examine your genitals. Check the front and sides of both legs starting with your thighs, all the way down to your ankles, tops of feet, between your toes, and under toenails. Don't forget to check the soles of your feet and heels.

Congratulations! You've just completed a procedure that could save your life!

Soothing Treatments
for Radiation Therapy

When my grandfather received radiation treatment for his facial basal cell carcinoma, the area became red and raw with blisters that stung and itched. His doctor gave him a gentle, bland ointment to apply to the affected area to soften his skin and reduce flaking of the surrounding dry, stiff tissue, thus soothing some of the irritation. If you're undergoing radiation therapy for skin cancer and have similar skin irritation as a result, there's a simple natural home remedy you can prepare to ease the symptoms. Mix evening primrose oil (enough to cover the affected area) with a drop of German chamomile essential oil, and apply topically 2 to 3 times a day. This treatment will help moisturize and heal the skin and reduce inflammation — although it's quite gentle, you should consult with your physician before using it.

Consulting the Experts

See an Esthetician If: Your esthetician is not the professional to see if you have skin cancer, but, if while performing a skin care procedure she happens to notice something that looks amiss, it is her responsibility to bring it to your attention and recommend that you see a dermatologist immediately.

See a Dermatologist If: If during your monthly self-examination you notice any skin changes of any kind, do not ignore the warning signs. Skin cancer is not always painful, but it can be dangerous. See your dermatologist immediately if you detect a suspicious spot.

CELLULITE

Cellulite is the dimpled, lumpy skin that most often appears on the thighs, hips, buttocks, and stomach. Cellulite is not a type of fat, but rather is a result of the relationship between skin and the fat layer beneath it. It affects women more than men because women tend to have more subcutaneous fat and slightly thinner skin.

Causes

If you were to ask ten different skin care and body-care experts, ranging from dermatologists to estheticians to massage therapists, to state the causes of cellulite, you'd get ten different answers. Here are some of the answers I received:

- There's no such thing as cellulite. It's just plain old fat. The cause is simply a lack of exercise and overeating.
- It's a result of stagnant circulation in various areas between the torso and the knees.
- Cellulite is a type of fat that traps extra water beneath the skin's surface, causing a puckered appearance.
- Cellulite is caused by toxins in the diet, such as artificial sweeteners, preservatives, and additives, which the body stores in fat cells.
- The appearance of cellulite is more apparent when the underlying muscle is untoned and flabby. In an athletic body the visible dimpling of the fat layer, if evident at all, is minimal.
- Cellulite is one of the side effects of a constipated colon and insufficient water intake, resulting in an overaccumulation of toxins. When toxins are not being released through the proper channels — the skin, kidneys, liver, and colon — they are stored in the fat tissue, isolated from the body and out of harm's way.
- Cellulite is a combination of fat, water, and wastes trapped beneath the skin in pockets within the connective fiber bands that hold the skin in place. As the amount of these materials increases, the pockets bulge, causing the familiar cottage-cheese effect.

All of these "causes" of cellulite ring true to a certain degree. Cellulite does consist of fatty tissue, water, and toxins, and the degree to which it affects you depends upon the types of food you consume as well as the amount and type of exercise you get. Although it can be difficult to eradicate, there are ways to eliminate it or at least minimize its appearance.

Preventing Cellulite Development

If you're one of the few people who isn't afflicted with cellulite, you're either very young or very fortunate. Even female
athletes who work out more than 2 hours a day can still have
a minor amount of cellulite on their thighs and buttocks. However, there are several lifestyle "adjustments" you can make —
if they're not already a part of your routine — that will not only
keep you healthier in general but will also help prevent the
formation of, or further development of, cellulite.

- ◆ Get up, move, and sweat! Daily, vigorous aerobic
  exercise is paramount, so fight your sedentary ten-
  dencies. Try jogging, walking, dancing, bicycling, or
  rollerblading to stimulate circulation throughout
  your body, especially from the waist down (the area
  most commonly affected by cellulite).
- ◆ Begin a regular weight-lifting routine to keep your
  underlying muscles toned and tight.
- ◆ Drink, drink, drink — water, that is. An ample intake of
  water will keep toxins flowing right out of your body.
- ◆ Eat a proper, balanced diet with as many whole,
  unrefined foods as possible.
- ◆ Avoid salty foods like the plague! Salt causes your
  body to retain water, which can exacerbate the
  appearance of cellulite.
- ◆ Stop smoking. Smoking impairs circulation and adds
  poisonous toxins to your bloodstream.
- ◆ Keep alcohol and caffeine consumption to a minimum. They contribute more toxins for your body to
  deal with, and they sap your body of valuable nutrients essential for skin health.
- ◆ Stay within your normal, healthy weight range. Cellulite is more pronounced if you are overweight.

Treatments for Cellulite

All professionals who treat cellulite agree upon one thing: Cellulite is a chronic condition that requires continual treatment
and maintenance. It is not a condition that you pay attention
to one day and not the next. As soon as you stop preventive

or treatment measures, cellulite will begin to build up again. To properly treat cellulite, you must make whatever method you decide upon a part of your regular routine.

The following treatment suggestions consist of diet and exercise programs. They really work for those who are motivated and diligent. You must be consistent in your efforts for smooth, tight, firm skin to prevail. Cellulite will respond positively to your new lifestyle habits, but it may be a long process. Remember, you didn't get into the shape you're in overnight — fat and cellulite will take just as long to disappear.

Please note, if you are overweight, I recommend a visit to your physician to alert her or him of your intention to begin a new diet and exercise program.

Aerobic weight lifting. This type of exercise combines the cardiovascular benefits of aerobics with strengthening and muscle-building weights. It makes you really sweat and seems to carve the fat right off my thighs and buttocks as fast as a hot knife through butter. When I'm consistent with this type of exercise, I usually see results in as little as 10 days. Unfortunately, very few workout tapes offer this type of exercise combination. Call your local gym to see if they offer classes.

Yoga. If you've never taken a yoga-for-strength class, you may think that yoga is for people who can't do strenuous exercise. That assumption couldn't be further from the truth. The practice of yoga consists of performing a series of postures that strengthen your muscles and joints using your own body weight for resistance. When you hold a pose, you're working your muscles isometrically (without moving). I find that yoga tones and elongates my muscles, making for a leaner, more lithe look. It builds balance, coordination, and strength, and is wonderfully de-stressing as well.

Dry brushing. This is a wonderful technique for improving skin tone, circulation, and lymph flow, and for shedding dry skin. See page 178 for how-to instructions.

Diet. Reduce your consumption of refined and simple carbohydrates, including white flour, sugar and sugar substitutes, chips, cake, cookies, crackers, popcorn, and french fries, to name a few. Such starchy, sugary foods offer minimal nutritional value and if eaten in excess, cause weight gain and water retention.

Anti-Cellulite Bath Treatment

The rosemary and lavender essential oils in this formula pamper and condition your skin, while the juniper and cypress essential oils exert a diuretic action, helping to reduce water retention. The salt aids in toxin elimination and muscle relaxation.

2 teaspoons (10 ml) almond, avocado, or sesame oil
1 teaspoon (5 ml) honey
1 teaspoon (5 ml) vodka, gin, or rum
2 drops juniper essential oil
3 drops cypress essential oil
4 drops lavender angustifolia essential oil
3 drops rosemary (chemotype linalol) essential oil
½ cup (125 ml) Epsom salts

To prepare the bath: Blend the oil, honey, alcohol, and essential oils in a small bowl. Set aside. Start the water running in the tub and add the salts; stir them around until they are dissolved. When the tub is full, pour in the oily mixture.

To use: Soak for approximately 20 minutes. Massage the cellulite-afflicted areas while you are soaking to help break down the fatty deposits. Then get out and briskly dry your skin using a thickly napped towel. Follow up with an application of body lotion to which you have added a drop of each of the essential oils in the ingredients list. You may partake of this bath up to 3 times a week.

Yield: 1 bath treatment

Consulting the Experts

See an Esthetician If: If you want to temporarily reduce the appearance of cellulite, your esthetician can help. She may offer an herbal body wrap treatment, which stimulates circulation, helps eliminate toxins and excess water, and revitalizes the skin's texture and tone. This is also a super way to relax. However, keep in mind that the small amount of weight shed, the tightening of the skin, and/or the inches lost are the result of water loss and will return within a day or two.

Estheticians who are trained in deep tissue massage may offer a series of anticellulite treatments. This requires that you receive an aggressive 1 hour massage (usually a lower body massage) 1 or 2 times a week, depending upon the severity of your condition, for a total of approximately eighteen treatments. The benefits include improved circulation and lymph flow, reduction of lactic acid, relaxed muscles, and improved skin texture. Following a massage, you may notice an increased need to urinate, as fluid has been pushed out of the subcutaneous tissues and must be eliminated. This fluid loss will result in a slight reduction in measurement. Maintenance services are required at the rate of one or two treatments a month thereafter. (Unfortunately, this can be quite time consuming and expensive.) Please note, if you have a heart condition, varicose veins, or diabetes, you should avoid this type of procedure.

See a Dermatologist If: If all your diligent effort in trying to reduce the amount of cellulite on your body has failed, your dermatologist may be of some assistance. A dermatologist can perform liposuction, a procedure in which a small suctioning device is inserted under the skin to remove fat cells. As wonderful and easy as it sounds, though, liposuction can be painful and expensive, and it may even worsen the dimpling and puckering symptoms in some patients. Not everyone is a good candidate for this type of surgery. Talk it over thoroughly with your doctor and discuss the pros and cons before deciding to undergo this surgical technique.

CHAPPED, DRY LIPS

You know what chapped lips feel like — dry, tight, flaky, cracked, and burning. All you want to do is lick them and put out the fire. Chapped lips are red or purplish in color and seem to absorb any moisture you put on them and then scream for more.

Causes of Chapped Lips

Your lips, unlike the rest of your skin, do not contain any sebaceous or sweat glands and therefore cannot moisturize themselves; they constantly need re-wetting. Normally, the small amount of saliva that reaches the surface of your lips via the tip of your tongue is sufficient to keep them moist. However, if the lip tissue is damaged from heat, cold, lipsticks, dry air, smoking, sunburn, herpes, infection, or topical or oral medications, your saliva will not be sufficient to prevent your lips from becoming dehydrated.

Prevention

Follow these simple tips to keep your smoocher soft and kissable:

- When venturing out into the sun, be it the beach or bright ski slope, don't forget to apply a lip balm with an SPF of 15 or higher. Lips can get sunburned, too!
- Brush your lips! After brushing your teeth, gently brush your lips as well. "Not only does it take away any chapping, but it plumps up the lip temporarily for that sought-after 'pouty' look," says Diane Irons, author of *The World's Best-Kept Beauty Secrets.*
- Apply a lip balm frequently throughout the day to create a moisture resistant barrier on your lips that will help prevent moisture loss.
- Keep hydrated! Drink lots of water throughout the day.
- Dab honey on your lips to soothe and protect. Honey acts as a humectant — it draws moisture from the air to your skin, thus keeping your lips soft and plump.
- Castor oil, the first ingredient in most lipsticks, can be applied straight out of the bottle for a glossy look.

Treatments for Chapped Lips

Chapped or chronically dry lips need constant moisture and protection from the elements. So pamper your lips with my delicious lip balm formula.

LIP SLICKER

5 tablespoons (75 ml) castor or jojoba oil (use
6 tablespoons [90 ml] if you prefer a thinner,
glossier texture)

1 tablespoon (15 ml) beeswax

1 teaspoon (5 ml) chopped alkanet root for deep red
color (optional)

1 teaspoon (5 ml) honey or vegetable glycerine

10 drops peppermint, orange, or lemongrass essential
oil for flavor

◆ **or** add 10 drops carrot seed essential oil to revi-
talize dry, chapped lip skin

◆ **or** add 10 drops of either tea tree or eucalyptus
essential oil for treatment of cold sores and
cracked, bleeding lips

To make:
1. Combine the oil and beeswax in a small saucepan
over low heat or in a double boiler and warm until the
wax is melted. Remove from heat.
2. If you desire a colorant, add alkanet root now and
let steep for 1 hour. Remelt oil and wax until liquid,
strain out alkanet, and proceed with the recipe.
3. While oil and wax mixture is still a warm liquid, add
honey or glycerine and essential oil(s), and blend the
mixture thoroughly. Pour into ¼–½ ounce (7–15 g) tins
or cosmetic jars while still hot. Will keep for up to 1
year or longer if refrigerated.
To use: Since a lip balm adds no moisture to your
lips, it is recommended that you provide moisture
first. Apply a drop of water or a dab of honey to the lip
surface and lightly pat with a tissue to remove the
excess. Then slather on a good layer of sweet or medicated lip balm to seal in the moisture you just
applied.
Yield: Approximately 3 ounces (90 g)

Consulting the Experts

See an Esthetician If: If you don't want to make your own lip-healing formula, your skin care professional will carry a tube or two of lip balm containing beeswax, castor oil, and/or vitamin E in her salon, though for the price, you can't beat making your own!

See a Dermatologist If: A common side effect of topical or oral prescription drugs, especially acne medications, is dry, tight, burning lips. If this occurs and the above recommendations don't provide enough relief, your physician might be able to recommend another medication or a remedy for the dryness.

COUPEROSE COMPLEXION

Couperose skin is highly sensitive facial skin characterized by dilated or expanded capillaries. A diffused redness, or erythema, is concentrated on the nose and cheeks. The capillaries can appear as tiny red dots or individual broken capillaries, or they can take on a spiderweb-like appearance, commonly called spider veins, a spider nevus, or spider telangiectasia. The tiny capillaries are quite visible through the skin's surface.

Causes of Couperose Skin

The classic appearance of couperose skin is, according to *Tabor's Cyclopedic Medical Dictionary,* "caused by capillary congestion, usually due to dilation of the superficial capillaries as a result of some nervous mechanism within the body, inflammation, or some external influence such as heat, sunburn, or cold." All skin types can suffer from a couperose condition, but those with fair skin and hair or sensitive, delicate, thin, or mature skin are most commonly affected. Smoking, excessive alcohol consumption, high blood pressure, temperature extremes, years of unprotected sun exposure, sunburn, and overzealous cleansing all contribute to couperose skin. Over the years vascular walls become damaged and can no longer handle the pressure of the blood flowing through them, so they break and leave you with a blotchy, ruddy complexion.

Prevention

Proper skin care is key to preventing the development or worsening of couperose skin. Wear sunscreen daily and avoid temperature extremes, or at least apply proper moisturizers prior to going outside. Avoid the causes of couperose skin listed above and pay attention to your health and stress level. It is amazing what nutritional neglect and environmental, work, and family stressors can do to your skin.

Furthermore, avoid alcohol-based toners, gritty facial scrubs, herbal steams, drying clay masks, and strong alpha-hydroxy and glycolic acid treatments, as these can be irritating if you suffer from this condition, even if it is just in its beginning stages.

Treatments

Couperose skin is a difficult condition to treat once it has developed, but with proper care you can help protect your skin against further deterioration and minimize the fragility of the capillaries.

Use gentle, mild products. You must use very gentle, fragrance- and color-free products to cleanse, tone, and moisturize. Lavender, rose, or German chamomile aromatic hydrosols make terrific anti-inflammatory and hydrating toners and aftershaves. They soothe the skin and reduce any feeling of surface dryness.

Exfoliate gently. Mix together equal parts of plain yogurt and finely ground sesame seed meal — 1 tablespoon (15 ml) is usually enough for one treatment. Gently massage the mixture onto your face, then rinse with cool water. This mild moisturizing and exfoliating mask is extremely gentle on the skin. It can be used once a week to clean fragile, sensitive skin and couperose complexions.

Supplement your diet. Increase your consumption of fresh, raw fruits and vegetables, especially those high in bioflavonoids (a class of phytochemicals found in the white inner rind of citrus fruits and in green and yellow vegetables, garlic, and onions). Bioflavonoids aid in strengthening capillary walls. Natural vitamin C with bioflavonoids might be a supplement to consider as well.

Consulting the Experts

See an Esthetician If: If you are in need of gentle, therapeutic cleansers and products to properly care for your couperose skin, your esthetician is the person to see. If you have couperose skin combined with another skin problem, she'll be able to guide you to the right product line.

See a Dermatologist If: If you'd like to eradicate those unsightly, red squiggly lines from your face, your dermatologist might recommend laser treatments to remove and destroy the defective surface capillaries.

CUTS, SCRAPES, AND OTHER IRRITATIONS

Let's face it — life can be hazardous! Everyday life is full of things that can bump, burn, scrape, grab, bruise, cut, bite, scratch, and poke your delicate skin. Minor injuries do and will happen, no matter where you are, leaving you with cuts, scrapes, and all sort of skin irritations.

Treatments for Irritations

Try these easy-to-make, natural remedies that will soothe irritations and help prevent infection.

Note: If you've stepped on a nail or received a puncture wound from any metallic element, be sure to get a tetanus shot right away.

INFECTION CORRECTION SKIN CLEANSER

After cleansing the wound with this infection fighter, follow with Calendula Ointment (see page 108) to help heal and relieve irritation.

 1 cup (250 ml) hydrogen peroxide
 20 drops tea tree essential oil
 20 drops spike lavender essential oil
 5 drops thyme (chemotype linalol) essential oil

To make: Combine all ingredients in an 8-ounce (250-ml) spray bottle or regular bottle, preferably glass. May store in a cool, dry cabinet for up to 1 year.
To use: Pour cool water over the affected area to clear it of debris, if necessary. Dab irritation with a cleanser-soaked cotton ball or gently pour the liquid directly onto the scrape, scratch, or insect bite. Use as needed to prevent infection, up to 3 times per day.
Yield: 1 cup (250 ml)

Consulting the Experts

See an Esthetician If: Everyday cuts and scrapes don't usually require the attention of a skin care specialist. However, if your esthetician carries a line of herb-based acne products, ask her if she sells a strong herbal astringent that contains either hydrogen peroxide or isopropyl alcohol. These particular products make good disinfectant washes and are handy to keep in first-aid kits.

See a Dermatologist If: If you notice that the affected area is not healing properly, or that it is red, sore, or filled with pus, you may have an infection. See your doctor as soon as possible to keep the infection from gettting any worse.

CALENDULA OINTMENT

This herbal ointment helps heal and relieve an amazing variety of skin irritations. In addition to soothing the usual assortment of cuts and abrasions, it makes an excellent preventive for diaper rash. Just apply to the little bottom after every diaper change to maintain fresh, healthy, soft skin. This ointment is also fabulous for dry, cracked hands and feet. Smells terrific, too!

½ cup (125 ml) all-vegetable shortening
10 drops calendula essential oil
10 drops everlasting or spike lavender essential oil
5 drops orange or lemon essential oil

To make: In a small bowl, allow the shortening to warm to room temperature. Add the essential oils. With a small whisk, whip ingredients together until thoroughly combined. Store in a glass or plastic container with a tight lid. Will keep, if refrigerated, for up to 1 year or up to 6 months if kept at room temperature.
To use: Clean the affected area and then apply the ointment. Use as necessary to help heal and prevent infection.
Yield: ½ cup (125 ml)

DERMATITIS

Dermatitis comes from the Latin *dermatos,* meaning "skin," and *itis,* meaning "inflammation." According to *Taber's Cyclopedic Medical Dictionary,* dermatitis is an "inflammation of the skin evidenced by itching, redness, and various skin lesions." These various skin lesions can include blisters, pimples, lumps, dry skin, and scales.

Causes of Dermatitis

Dermatitis generally falls under one of two categories: irritant or allergic. *Irritant contact dermatitis,* the most common, can result in stinging, itching, redness, or burning sensations. It is an inflammation of the skin caused by contact with irritants to which you may be sensitive, such as abrasive cleansers, hair dyes, eye shadow, mascara, bar soaps, deodorants, moisturizers, wool fabrics, nickel (in jewelry), plant sap, and latex gloves. Construction workers frequently complain of rough, red, sore hands because they handle a variety of irritants — cement mix, fiberglass, acids, wood and metal chemicals, and paint, to name a few — and are at risk for developing *occupational contact dermatitis.* Health-care workers, who frequently wash their hands, are at risk from constant exposure to water and detergents.

Allergic contact dermatitis is an inflammation of the skin that can result in swelling, redness, itching, hives, and oozing blisters, and is caused by a specific ingredient in a product to which you are allergic, such as lanolin, artificial colors, preservatives, fragrances, medicated creams, rubber, and glues. Upon your first contact with the potential allergen, a reaction is rare. However, repeated exposure will cause a reaction to occur even if the level of contact with the allergen is very low. This type of dermatitis has a tendency to spread to other parts of the body, away from the original contact site.

Prevention

If you are prone to allergies, and unsure of your reaction to a skin care product, try to find a tester bottle and place a little on your wrist or inner upper arm and leave it there for 8 to 12 hours. If all is still well, then you can generally feel safe about that product. Many times, though, it is not possible to test a product or item first, so proceed with caution. Take heart — most people can use common, everyday items without a problem, but if you're a sensitive type, take time to read labels and educate yourself about ingredients. Buy color-free, fragrance-free, and chemical-free products when available.

SKINFORMATION

Fragrance additives, whether natural or synthetic, cause more allergic contact dermatitis than any other ingredient. Preservatives are the second most common cause.

Treatments for Dermatitis

The symptoms of dermatitis can be quite irritating and annoying, so for temporary relief while your skin is healing, try the Comfrey Comfort Spray, a cooling, soothing, herbal anti-inflammatory formula.

COMFREY COMFORT SPRAY

Comfrey acts as an emollient, softening and comforting your skin. The peppermint and eucalyptus essential oils add a cooling quality to the spray.

1 cup (250 ml) distilled water
1 teaspoon (5 ml) dried, chopped comfrey root, or 1 tablespoon (15 ml) fresh, chopped root
½ cup (125 ml) aloe vera juice
10 drops calendula essential oil
10 drops German chamomile essential oil
2 drops peppermint essential oil (optional)
2 drops eucalyptus essential oil (optional)

To make: In a small saucepan, bring water to a boil. Add the comfrey root, then reduce heat and simmer, covered, to allow herb to decoct for 30 minutes. Strain into a small bowl. Add aloe vera juice and essential oils. Stir thoroughly. Pour liquid into a 12-ounce (375-ml) spray bottle or divide into two smaller bottles. If refrigerated, the spray will keep for approximately 2 weeks. If refrigeration is not possible, store in cool location and discard after 1 week.

To use: Shake well before each use and spray as often as necessary onto inflamed, itchy, burning, irritated areas.

Yield: 1½ cups (375 ml)

Consulting the Experts

See an Esthetician If: If you are reacting to a cosmetic product recommended by your esthetician, let her know. Sometimes she can return it to the manufacturer and refund your money. She'll also want to note your reaction in her records and may ask that you come in so that she can examine the irritated area and apply a soothing, anti-inflammatory treatment free of charge to ease your discomfort.

See a Dermatologist If: Dermatitis will usually clear up on its own once the irritant is removed, but if your dermatitis is not responding to home treatment, your doctor may wish to prescribe a cortisone or hydrocortisone lotion for short-term use. Antibiotics may be necessary if infection has set in.

DRY, FLAKY SKIN

Does your skin have small pores and a fine, thin texture? Does it soak up moisturizer like a sponge and keep begging for more? Does it get tight right after cleansing? Does it tend to become scaly, itchy, flaky, hot, red, sensitive to the touch, or parched? Well, my friend, you have dry skin, and this skin type ages faster than any other. Just what you wanted to hear, right?

Causes of Dry Skin

There are basically three types of dry skin: oil dry, water dry or dehydrated, and mature or aging skin. Oil-dry skin is caused by sebaceous glands that aren't functioning properly. Either they're lazy and sluggish or are simply failing to produce ample sebum. This type of dryness is usually inherited. Water-dry or dehydrated skin may be producing a sufficient amount of sebum but it's still dry on the surface due to a lack of moisture or water or as a side effect of medication. The third type of dry skin is caused by the natural aging process — a natural slowdown in the skin's regenerative capabilities. It just doesn't produce skin-softening sebum in the quantities that it did when it was younger.

Prevention

While you may not be able to prevent dry skin from occurring entirely, you can help keep it at bay by following these tips:

Avoid caffeine, smoking, and alcohol. They act as diuretics and are guaranteed to suck you dry.

Increase your water level. Drink up! Make sure to drink at least eight glasses of pure water a day to keep your skin and body properly hydrated. Drink more if you're super active.

Add oil to your bath. Add a tablespoon (15 ml) or so of almond, jojoba, olive, or hazelnut oil to your bath water after you've soaked for about 5 minutes. By soaking first, your skin gets plumped up by the water, then by adding the oil, it will seal in the absorbed moisture.

Protect your skin from the elements. Wind, sun, heat, cold, and dry office and airplane air can quickly cause or exacerbate the condition of dry skin. Apply a moisturizer before exposing your skin to these moisture-sapping villains. A lavender, rose, or German chamomile aromatic hydrosol sprayed onto your face, neck, hair, chest, and hands helps to keep your skin wonderfully refreshed and hydrated.

Limit hot water contact. Avoid long, hot showers and baths, especially during cold weather, as they dehydrate the skin. Warm showers and baths of short duration, though, are beneficial to dry skin. Also, limit bathing or washing your face to once a day, usually right before you retire. When you arise, apply a bit of herbal facial splash or toner or spritz your face (and body, if it needs treatment as well) with an aromatic hydrosol and you're ready to go.

Increase EFAs in your diet. Chow down on salmon, herring, mackerel, bluefish, and sardines. These cold-water fish are a rich source of omega-3 fatty acids, which can help replace moisture in dry hair and skin. Also consider adding evening primrose oil to your diet. I take one 1,300 mg capsule daily — or every other day, depending on my body's needs — and my skin just blooms! Flaxseed oil supplementation is also beneficial — 1 tablespoon (15 ml) is the standard recommended dosage.

Buy humidifiers. They work wonders in restoring healthful humidity to your dry home or office environment.

Use only gentle cleansers. Avoid cleansers such as deodorant soaps and harsh abrasives. These can cause your skin to feel like a dried-out Thanksgiving turkey. Use a moisturizing soap, soap-free products, or a gentle grain-based cleanser.

Treatments for Dry Skin

Most dermatologists recommend plain old petroleum jelly as an effective barrier against moisture loss. It's messy, but it works. If you're adverse to applying petroleum products to your skin, try a nonpetroleum jelly product available in health food stores.

GIVE DRY SKIN THE ONE-TWO KNOCKOUT

Perform these two treatments as often as 3 times per week.

Step 1: Exfoliate. This should always be the first step toward healing dry skin. Dead surface skin cells can, over time, build up and become unresponsive to lotions and creams. In order for your moisturizer to do its job, you must first get rid of this dead barrier. I like to use a gentle, grain-based scrub for my face. Mix 1 teaspoon (5 ml) ground oatmeal, 1 teaspoon (5 ml) white cosmetic clay, and 1 teaspoon (5 ml) ground flaxseed in a small bowl and add a bit of whole milk or cream. Stir everything together until a smooth paste forms and apply this to your face, gently massaging in a circular motion for about 1 minute. Rinse, and pat dry.

For my body I make a scrub that's a bit more abrasive. Combine 1–2 tablespoons (15–30 ml) salt with 1–2 tablespoons (15–30 ml) olive or quality vegetable oil in a small bowl. While in the shower, thoroughly scrub your entire body, making sure to spend a little extra time on the soles of the feet. Rinse and pat dry.

Step 2: Moisturize. After you've exfoliated, you're ready for moisture. Apply your favorite moisturizer to your face and body, or try good old vegetable shortening. (Shortening is typically made from 100 percent soybean oil and it soaks in rapidly — if you don't apply too much, that is!) I usually put my flannel gown and socks on after this and go to bed. You'll awaken with gloriously, soft, smooth skin.

Consulting the Experts

See an Esthetician If: Your esthetician can tell you if your skin is oil dry or dehydrated and recommend treatment plans to bring it into balance. She is also a good source for gentle exfoliating creams and scrubs if you'd rather purchase them than make your own.

See a Dermatologist If: Generally a dry skin condition is relatively easy to remedy, but if you've tried everything to alleviate your dry skin and it's still not responding, perhaps you have something more serious and a visit to your doctor might prove prudent.

ECZEMA

Atopic dermatitis or atopic eczema, commonly referred to as simply eczema, usually begins in childhood and is hereditary. It mainly affects young children, teens, and young adults and is typically seen in families with a history of hay fever, asthma, or other allergies.

One of the early signs of infantile eczema is a localized, raised rash and swelling. As the disease progresses, redness and small blisters or vesicles form that can, over time, begin to ooze and crust. After age two, many children improve dramatically and have very few symptoms. That's good news, as

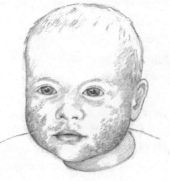

In infants, eczema is usually characterized by a localized, raised red rash on the face, elbows, or knees.

infantile eczema can be hard on both the child and the parents — all the child wants to do is scratch, and so becomes irritable and unable to sleep; all the parents want to do is help their child and get some needed rest!

Eczema is not limited to childhood, though. It may go away temporarily and then flare up later in life. It may fluctuate seasonally as well. Eczema in adults tends to be dry, red to brownish gray, thickened, scaly skin. Intense itching causes some people to scratch until they bleed, which leads to infection, oozing, and crusting.

In infants, the skin rash usually begins on the face, elbows, or knees and may spread to other areas. Later in life, it can affect the elbow and knee folds, hands, ankles, wrists, neck, and upper chest.

SKINFORMATION

According to the National Eczema Association for Science and Education, "Individuals with atopic dermatitis have a lifelong tendency to suffer from various health problems:

- Dry, easily irritated skin
- Occupational skin disease — particularly hand dermatitis, causing considerable work loss
- Skin infections, especially staph and herpes
- Eye problems — cataracts and eyelid dermatitis
- Psychological disruption of family and social relationships

Causes of Eczema

The cause is actually unknown, but rest assured, eczema is not contagious. There are, however, many stressors or trigger factors that can aggravate the condition. These include cold weather, dry winter house heat and raw winter wind, emotional and physical stress, wool clothing, chafing from clothing, detergents, solvents, perfumes, dyes, heat and sweating, athlete's foot, herpes, pet dander, pollen, and food allergens.

Prevention

Here are a few tips to help prevent eczema flare-ups:

Moisturize, moisturize, moisturize! Unlike moist, soft, and flexible skin, dry skin is brittle and prone to cracking and infection, so keep your skin intact and your effective barrier healthy. Never let your skin dry out! Infused calendula oil (page 139) makes a particularly effective and soothing body moisturizer — massage into commonly affected areas as often as necessary.

Relax. Recognize your stressors, whatever they may be — work, family life, school, finances, or others — and learn to effectively manage them. The common reaction to stress in people prone to atopic dermatitis is red flushing and itching.

Know your genes. If eczema tends to run in your family, be prepared. Eat healthy, drink healthful immune strengthening herb teas (see Skin Ailment Assailment recipe, page 142), and avoid anything that can be a detriment to your health — smoking, lack of exercise, stress, soda, coffee, junk food, alcohol, and aggravating people and situations.

Supplement your diet. You need adequate intake of essential fatty acids and vitamins E and A to help keep your skin moisturized from within and win the battle against external dryness. In addition, make sure you are getting a good daily dose of vitamins C and B; zinc; and quercetin, a flavonoid, which may help prevent the formation of skin rashes.

Drink lots of fluids. Once again, I must reiterate: be sure to drink plenty of fluids, especially water and fresh fruit and vegetable juices to keep your body hydrated.

Treatments for Eczema

If you are fortunate enough to live near the ocean, take advantage of the healing properties of salt water. The cool ocean water will help relieve itching, inflammation, and general irritation caused by many forms of dermatitis, including eczema.

Evening primrose oil. According to Erica Lewis, author of "Essential Fatty Acids" in the July 1998 issue of *Les Nouvelles Esthetiques,* "Those with eczema may have an essential fatty acid deficiency. It is important for eczema sufferers to boost their dietary intake of the essential fatty acids because EFAs plump up the cell membranes and help repair old membranes and construct new ones. Eczema, psoriasis, dandruff, hair loss, dryness, and brittle nails respond to EFAs added to the diet."

Ocean Potion

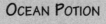

Landlocked readers for whom the ocean is just a distant summer's memory can enjoy a sea salt bath at home. If your eczema is weeping, oozing, and crusting, this treatment will help to soothe and cleanse the affected area(s), drain any infected sites, and aid in healing.

> 1 cup (250 ml) sea salt
> 5 drops carrot seed essential oil
> 5 drops calendula essential oil
> 2 teaspoons (10 ml) almond oil
> 1 tablespoon (15 ml) vodka, rum, or gin

To make: As the water runs into the tub, pour in the sea salt to dissolve. As the tub is filling, combine the oils and alcohol in a small bowl, stirring rapidly to blend. Set aside.

To use: Soak in the tub for 5–10 minutes to allow your skin to absorb moisture, then add the oils and alcohol and swish them throughout the water with your hands. These ingredients will soften and condition your skin. Soak for 10–15 minutes longer, then pat dry and apply your favorite cream or lotion to seal in vital moisture. *Note:* Don't soak for longer than 20 minutes and only use warm water, as hot water will actually dehydrate your skin.

Yield: 1 treatment

Clinical research has shown that evening primrose oil helps many people with arthritis pain, skin disorders, asthma, allergies, heart disease, and eczema. This seed oil is high in gamma-linolenic acid (GLA), an essential fatty acid that is needed by the body to produce the anti-inflammatory prostaglandins believed to combat these diseases and in turn strengthen cell membrane layers. Dosage recommendations range from 500 mg up to 3 to 4 grams per day, depending on the severity of the condition. Consult with your physician to find the right dosage for your particular situation.

Moisturizing treatments. With eczema, you must keep moisture in. Apply a good moisturizer immediately after showering or bathing. I recommend mixing vegetable shortening or a nonpetroleum jelly with a drop or two of lavender, calendula, German chamomile, or carrot seed essential oil and massaging the mixture onto your entire body. You can also use it to spot treat as necessary. This application creates a barrier to hold moisture in your skin that will help prevent further drying and itching of your eczema.

SOOTHING LICORICE TEA

In cases of skin irritations, including eczema, licorice can act as an anti-inflammatory agent upon the skin.

2 tablespoons (60 ml) dried licorice root
6 cups (1,500 ml) water

To make: Place the licorice and water in a saucepan, cover, and bring to a boil. Reduce heat and gently simmer, still covered, for 40 minutes. Strain.
To use: To relieve itching and irritation, add to a tub full of warm (not hot) water and soak for 10–15 minutes. You can also dab the tea directly onto itchy, dry patches of skin several times daily.
Yield: 6 cups, or 1 bath treatment

Another moisturizing treatment for irritated skin is to add ½ to 1 cup (125–250 ml) of finely ground or colloidal oatmeal to tepid bath water and have a good soak. This old-fashioned bath remedy is good for all types of dermatitis. A few cups of Soothing Licorice Tea (see page 119) added to bath water will also help relieve itching.

Consulting the Experts

See an Esthetician If: Your esthetician should carry a quality line of skin-enriching creams that will help seal in vital moisture and keep itching at bay. She may recommend a mild exfoliating gel to aid in gently removing the dead skin buildup that makes eczema unsightly.

See a Dermatologist If: If your eczema is not responding to home treatment, you may need to seek a doctor's advice. Medications such as topical or oral cortisone and antihistamines to control the itching are frequently useful for symptomatic relief, preferably as short-term treatments, as these drugs have undesirable side effects.

Another avenue to investigate is homeopathic medicine. Diseases such as arthritis, eczema, and psoriasis often respond positively to this type of complementary treatment. I highly recommend reading *Healing with Homeopathy*, by Dr. Wayne Jonas and Dr. Jennifer Jacobs.

TIRED EYES

Are you a sight for sore eyes, or are your sore eyes a sight? Stressed eyes can be dry, itchy, irritated, red, burning, tired, or watery, and occasionally are surrounded by puffiness and dark circles. Sometimes these windows to your soul need a little pick-me-up. The treatments that follow should put the sparkle back.

Causes of Tired Eyes

Want to know a guaranteed way to look older quickly? Neglect your health and stress yourself out! Your eyes reflect the real you — a partier, an outdoors person, a sun worshiper, or a workaholic — and are the first part of your complexion to show signs of aging. The skin directly beneath the eyes does not contain sebaceous glands to lubricate it and is so very thin that a little neglect will immediately be reflected in and around your pretty peepers.

Many factors contribute to visual stress and unsightly eyes. A poor diet rich in simple carbohydrates and salt such as snack chips, candy, and fast food has a tendency to cause fluid retention in the eye area, and does nothing to nourish the rest of your body. Stress, lack of sleep, fluorescent light, dim light, sun, injury, alcohol, smoking, dry air, swimming in chlorinated pools, watching television, cosmetic fragrances, allergies, medication, repeated friction (such as eye makeup removal or contact lens placement), and sickness can lead to irritation, eye strain, dark circles, fine lines, and crow's-feet.

Dark circles, in particular, trouble many men and women. They make you look sick, tired, and older than your years. "In order to correct the problem of dark circles and other blemishes," states Dr. Victor Beraja, a board-certified plastic surgeon and author of "Eliminating Dark Eye Circles" (*Les Nouvelles Esthetiques,* March 1998), "one must know that cells beneath the epidermis called melanocytes produce the pigment that forms dark circles . . . when stimulated by a wide range of things, including . . . the gentle pull on the lids to insert contact lenses. . . . When this is repeated on a daily basis, for a long period of time, it can cause hyperpigmentation. Allergies and dry eyes work in a similar way. Irritation caused by these conditions lead a person to rub their eyes which again can cause hyperpigmentation. If the skin is excessively dry or sensitive to sun, even short exposure to the sun will irritate and stimulate the production of pigment. Of course, not all dark circles are caused by hyperpigmentation. Some circles are caused by swelling, poor circulation, and fluid retention."

Dark circles can also be the result of venous circulation, which is partially visible through the extremely thin skin beneath the eyes. Neither bleaching nor herbal treatments will work if this is the cause. You best bet is makeup!

Prevention

To prevent the unsightly appearance of red, irritated eyes and dark circles, try these tips:

Wear sunscreen. Always wear sunscreen, either by itself or under your makeup — every day! Sunscreen helps prevent melanin formation within the thin, delicate skin around your eyes. Melanin is the dark pigment that can show up as unsightly dark circles.

Treat them gently. Don't pull or rub your eyes. Take eye makeup off gently using vegetable oil or a product specifically made to dissolve this type of makeup. Avoid using petroleum jelly or heavy cream near your eyes, as these can block the tear ducts and lead to water retention and puffy eyes.

Moisturize. Apply a water-based lotion or gel around the eye area once every day after cleansing to moisturize the delicate skin.

Take a break. Are you stuck behind a glaring computer screen or do you sit behind a desk grading papers or crunching numbers, all the while squinting your eyes? Give your eyes a break. Hour after hour of looking in one direction at small print and computer-screen light leads to eye irritation, tiredness, headache, and lazy eyes. Periodically stand up, stretch, and, ideally looking out a window, focus on something far in the distance, preferably a beautiful green tree or mountains. Without turning your head, look side to side several times, then up and down. Now, don't your eyes feel better?

Tune out. Don't be a TV addict. The glare from the screen is not good for your eyes.

Sleep. Pep up with plenty of sound sleep — one of the best eye (and body) beautifiers there is!

Treatments for Tired Eyes

Hydrosol spritzer. I sit at my computer writing for hours at a time and frequently get sore, dry, irritated eyes. My favorite treatment is to keep a bottle of lavender hydrosol (available from Simplers Botanical Company) handy and spritz my face and eyes with it as often as necessary. The liquid is so pure and gentle that I can spray it directly into my opened eyes. I find it extremely soothing. German chamomile and rose hydrosol work equally well.

Milk. For swollen eyelids, dip cotton balls or cosmetic squares into icy cold whole milk. Lie down, and apply soaked cotton to swollen eyelids and leave on for 5 to 10 minutes. The high fat content of whole milk provides a moisturizing treatment for the delicate, thin skin around your eyes.

Herbal compresses. My herbalist friend, Jean Argus, owner of Jean's Greens (see resources), makes a delightfully refreshing herbal tea mixture called "For Your Eyes Only," containing eyebright, bilberry, chickweed, calendula, lavender, and goldenseal leaf. It's available in tea bags, which can be moistened with cool water and applied to irritated eyes, or made into an infusion to use an eyewash or simply enjoyed as a nourishing beverage for your body.

You can make your own herbal compress with calendula or lavender using the Soothing Eye Compress recipe.

SOOTHING EYE COMPRESS

2 cups (500 ml) water
4 teaspoons (20 ml) freshly picked calendula flower
   petals or lavender buds (or 2 teaspoons [10 ml] dried)
Cosmetic cotton squares or large cotton balls

To make: Bring the water to a boil. Remove from heat, add the flowers, and cover. Steep for 15 minutes, then place in the refrigerator and allow to cool for 1 hour. Strain. Keep refrigerated and use within 4 days.

To use: Moisten four cotton squares or balls with the herbal tea, squeezing out any excess liquid. Lie down and place the cotton over your eyes — two pieces for each. Leave on for 5–10 minutes.

Yield: 6–8 treatments

HERBAL EYEWASH

In her book, *The Herbal Medicine Cabinet,* published by Celestial Arts Press (Berkeley, CA: 1998), Master Herbalist Debra St. Claire recommends this recipe for general eye care. "This eyewash is for tired, strained eyes. It cleanses the tear ducts and stimulates circulation, which contributes to the tea's fame as a vision restorative." The eyewash should be made fresh for each treatment as it does not store well in the refrigerator.

> 1 cup (250 ml) distilled water
> 1 tablespoon (15 ml) dried eyebright
> Glass eyecup (available in pharmacies)

To make:
1. In a small saucepan, bring the water to a boil, then remove from heat. Add the eyebright, cover, and let steep, for 10 minutes.
2. While the eyewash is steeping, sterilize a glass eyecup by submerging it in boiling water for 5 minutes.
3. Strain the tea through a paper towel or doubled cotton cloth into a glass measuring cup. Cool until the tea is lukewarm.
To use: Fill the eyecup with the cooled solution, pouring from the measuring cup into the eyecup (as opposed to dipping the eyecup in the solution). Bend your head forward, place the eyecup firmly on your eye, then tip your head back, letting the solution wash the eye as you blink several times. It is helpful to hold a folded paper towel against your cheek to catch any drips. Discard the used solution and refill the eyecup. Repeat the application to the same eye 3 separate times. Then resterilize the eyecup (this will prevent contamination of the second eye) and repeat the procedure on the other eye.
Yield: 1 treatment

Tea. To reduce puffiness around the eyes, brew some regular black or green tea. They contain tannin, a natural astringent that helps to reduce swelling and puffiness. Chill the tea bags. Lie down with your head slightly elevated above your body and apply tea bags to your eyes. Rest with tea bags over closed eyes for approximately 20 minutes.

Fluid intake. Swollen eyes and dark circles can sometimes be the result of toxin buildup in the body as well as dehydration. Be sure to drink plenty of water daily in order to flush toxins and excess sodium from your body. When the body is dehydrated, the kidneys try to retain water, which results in puffiness and general ill health. The more water you drink, the less you will retain — it's a fact!

Over-the-counter products. Over-the-counter products containing skin-lightening hydroquinone or natural kojic acid have been proven effective in lightening hyperpigmented circles (those that are not hereditary) beneath the eyes. *Caution:* Always read the label of an over-the-counter product and make sure it specifically says that the product can be used around the eyes, as these creams can be quite irritating to some skin types, especially around the delicate eye area.

Consulting the Experts

See an Esthetician If: Your esthetician should be able to offer a few soothing eye treatments and recommend daily hydrating gels and light creams to ease the appearance of fine lines and wrinkles. Ask her if she offers a gentle exfoliating treatment to help lighten dark pigmentation under the eyes. If all else fails, I'm sure she be glad to sell you a quality makeup concealer to cover up your troubles!

See a Dermatologist If: If home remedies or a visit to your esthetician don't help soothe and beautify your eyes, then a visit to your dermatologist or eyecare specialist may be in order. Swelling, vision disorders, soreness, headaches, the feeling of roughness in your eyes when you blink, or watery eyes may be signs of internal problems or allergies.

HERPES SIMPLEX TYPE I

Herpes manifests as burning, tingling, itching, red, uncomfortable, tender blisters that appear on the lips and face. Some blisters are the size of pinheads and others may develop into much larger sores. The blisters begin to heal and form yellowish hard crusts, usually within a few days. Eventually this crust falls off and leaves the skin unscarred.

Causes

There are two types of the herpes simplex virus: HSV Type I, which most of us are familiar with, causes what is often called a cold sore or fever blister. HSV Type II causes genital sores and can be quite painful. I will discuss HSV Type I only.

Contrary to what their common names imply, cold sores and fever blisters are not caused by colds or fevers. Rather, they're caused by one of a group of viruses that is responsible for a number of other maladies such as mononucleosis, shingles, and chicken pox. Over 50 percent of the American population carry some form of the herpes virus in their nerve cells, where it quietly rests until set off by stress or illness.

SKINFORMATION

According to the American Academy of Dermatology, between 200,000 and 500,000 persons "catch" genital herpes each year and the number of Type I infections is many times higher. Prevention of this disease, which is contagious before and during an outbreak, is important.

Prevention

Here are some tips to help prevent this pesky virus from catching a foothold in your system:

Avoid undue stress. Flare-ups frequently occur when life is full of stressors from work, family, relationships, excessive heat and sunlight, illness, gastrointestinal upset, or respiratory infection. Anything that compromises the immune system can trigger a herpes outbreak.

Avoid spreading the contagion. To avoid catching or spreading the disease, do not kiss an infected person or kiss anyone while you are infected. Also, avoid sharing cups, eating utensils, or cosmetics and sexual contact with anyone that you suspect is infected.

Dry them out. If you're already infected, prevent a painful secondary infection. Don't get the sores wet, don't touch and pick at them, and don't cover them with bandages. They need to dry out, not be kept moist.

Treatments for Herpes

Currently, there is nothing that can totally prevent future herpes outbreaks and cure the underlying cause of the disease. All treatments are for symptomatic relief. There are several over-the-counter HSV Type I treatments to choose from. These formulations will usually relieve the pain, cool the burning, and aid in healing. Most come in either a lip balm or gel form; the active ingredients are generally phenol, camphor, menthol, and eucalyptus.

Soothing teas. Cold, strong lemon balm or peppermint tea can be applied to blisters that are inflamed and/or burning to help ease the pain and reduce the heat.

Supplement your diet. From a nutritional standpoint, the essential amino acid lysine has been shown to inhibit the growth of the herpes virus. Five hundred milligrams daily of lysine (available in most health food stores) is the common dosage taken between flare-ups with higher amounts taken during an outbreak. Lysine therapy does not have any side effects, but it would be prudent to check with your health professional first before adding it in supplement form to your diet. Some of the best food sources of lysine include salmon, canned fish, beef, goat and cow's milk, cooked mung beans, cheese, beans, cottage cheese, brewer's yeast, and shellfish.

On the other hand, the nonessential amino acid arginine has been shown to stimulate the growth of the virus. Arginine

HERPES HEALING DROPS

To speed healing and help dry up oozing blisters, these antiviral herbal essential oil drops should provide relief.

2 tablespoons (30 ml) almond, jojoba, avocado, hazelnut, or soybean oil
2 drops blue cypress essential oil
2 drops peppermint essential oil
2 drops oregano essential oil
2 drops tea tree essential oil
2 drops eucalyptus essential oil

To make: To a 1-ounce (30-ml) glass bottle, add all ingredients and shake vigorously. Allow oils to blend for 24 hours prior to use. Store bottle in a cool, dry place for up to 1 year.

To use: Apply the mixture by the drop, up to 3 times per day, to affected areas and gently massage into skin. Avoid ingesting this blend — do not let it drip into your mouth.

Yield: Approximately 1 ounce (30 ml)

foods to avoid if you are prone to herpes outbreaks are: peanut butter, gelatin, chocolate, various nuts and seeds, and some cereals. Purchase a good nutrition guide so that you can educate yourself as to what foods are best to consume.

Support your immune system. Foods high in vitamins A, B, and C, zinc, and flaxseed oil all support immune system function and are beneficial to those suffering from HSV Type I.

Consulting the Experts

See an Esthetician If: Your esthetician may carry a good-quality herbal medicated lip balm specifically for minor cold sores or may be able to recommend a product — give her a call!

See a Dermatologist If: If you suffer from recurrent or severe Herpes Type I or II breakouts, your doctor may want to prescribe oral antiviral medications to reduce the number of attacks. Try to find a nutritionally oriented dermatologist who is familiar with complementary herpes treatments so that you may avoid drug usage if possible.

HIVES

I have a close friend who has a classic Type A personality. She works at two high-stress jobs a total of 60 to 70 hours per week, is a perfectionist, drinks an average of 5 cups of coffee a day, and teaches karate for 2 hours, 3 nights a week.

One summer day in 1996, during a very stressful and emotional period at her primary job, she began to develop intense itching on her torso, then on her neck and chest. The following day she woke up covered in roundish, red, raised blotches. She had no idea what was going on. Upon showing her husband her skin condition, he calmly told her she had a case of hives, commonly known as urticaria. She visited a dermatologist who confirmed the diagnosis.

Since then, whenever my friend finds herself under a heavy stress load, the itching begins and within minutes the pink swellings or wheals, as they are called, develop and last about 30 minutes, then disappear just as suddenly.

Hives can vary in size from as small as a pea to as large as 10 inches (25 cm) in diameter, usually itch, burn, or sting as they form, and fade away without a trace.

Causes of Hives

Angioedema, or hives that form around the lips, eyes, or genitals, generally result in excessive swelling, but tend to disappear within 24 hours. *Acute urticaria* is a term used to describe hives that last less than 6 weeks. This is the most common type of hives and usually appear in response to a food or drug allergy or infection. Hives that are caused by a food or drug allergy can, in addition to manifesting on the skin, result in the release of large amounts of histamines. Histamines are natural chemicals located in the skin that, when activated by an injury, allergic reaction, or other stressor, can cause flushing of the skin, swelling, tightness in the chest, wheezing, and a feeling of faintness. *Chronic urticaria* refers to outbreaks lasting for more than 6 weeks. Their cause is more difficult to pinpoint.

Physical urticarias are hives that develop from pressure, insect bites, vibration, cold, heat, exercise, or sunlight. *Solar urticaria* is a rare disorder in which hives develop within minutes after exposure to the sun, but disappear within hours.

Prevention

Hives are a very common malady, affecting approximately 10 to 20 percent of the population with at least one bout in their lifetime. Prevention can be difficult because you never know if you will be allergic to a new food or drug or if a new stressful situation in your life will cause hives. The best preventive is to avoid foods and drugs that are known systemic irritants and to minimize stress in your life.

Treatments for Hives

Find the cause, then eliminate it. According to dermatologists, this is the best treatment for hives. Unfortunately, this is not always the easiest of tasks to accomplish.

Soothing treatments. Treatments such as ice or cold aloe vera gel compresses can be applied directly to hives to help relieve the itching, shrink the wheals, and block the further release of histamines into your skin. One cup (250 ml) of baking soda and a few drops of lavender essential oil added to bath water will make a skin-relieving soak.

Relaxation therapy. In whatever form you seek — exercise, meditation, reiki, massage, reflexology, painting — relaxation therapy will aid in stress reduction, which is key to managing stress-induced hives.

Elimination diet. An elimination diet, guided by your doctor, nutritionist, or naturopath, can help to determine a particular food allergy and prevent future outbreaks of food-induced hives.

Supplement your diet. Vitamin C acts as a natural antihistamine, so make sure your diet includes ample amounts. You may want to supplement with 1,000 mg daily during an episode to help reduce the swelling.

Consulting the Experts

See an Esthetician If: If you need to unload the day's stresses, book a facial or body treatment with your esthetician. An hour in her chair or on her treatment table will do wonders for your nerves. Ask her to add a few drops of lavender or German chamomile essential oil to her massage cream or perhaps to a mask and breathe deeply of the relaxing aroma.

If you have hives at the time of your appointment, ask her if she can apply a cold compress with a few drops German chamomile essential oil to help reduce the inflammation and relieve the itching.

See a Dermatologist If: An acute skin reaction to a food or drug can be life-threatening. If breathing becomes impaired, seek out emergency room treatment immediately. If you are having difficulty locating the cause of your hives, your doctor or naturopath may want to question you about food or drug allergies. Additionally, there are a number of infections that can cause hives, and these need to be ruled out as well. For temporary relief, antihistamines can ease minor swelling and itching, but severe, recurrent hives may require an injection of epinephrine (adrenaline) or a topical cortisone cream. Remember, the best possible course of treatment is to find the root cause of the hives and eliminate it, not to have to depend on drug therapy.

HYPERPIGMENTATION

"Out, out damned spot!" If only that's all it took — three magic words and those pesky skin discolorations would disappear forever. I'm afraid it's not that simple. You know what I'm talking about here — those flat, roundish, noncarcinogenic brown or reddish brown spots that, the older you get, frequently develop on the hands, arms, face, shoulders, feet, and legs. They're mainly a cosmetic, not health, concern.

Causes

Epidermal hyperpigmentation is the result of excess pigmentation, or melanin accumulation, in the epidermal or dermal layer, and it is a harmless condition. Age, sun exposure, pregnancy, birth control pills, injury, chicken pox, shingles, acne scars, and heredity all play a role in the formation of hyperpigmented areas.

Chloasma gravidarum, or pregnancy mask, as it is commonly called, appears as brownish pigmentation areas on the face and neck. This uneven skin tone, due to fluctuating hormones and heightened sun sensitivity, usually disappears after delivery as the hormones settle back down.

Age spots or liver spots, also called lentigines, are caused by accumulated sun damage and may begin to appear in your thirties, depending upon the extent of past sun exposure. These discolorations often do not respond to commercial fade creams, but can be removed by your dermatologist if they really bother you.

Freckles are usually hereditary, can appear anywhere on the body, often darken with sun exposure, but tend to fade if you stay out of the sun. As a child, my cheeks and nose used to be covered with freckles, but now they've completely disappeared.

The skin on your pressure points, such as the elbows, knees, knuckles, palms, and soles of your feet, also tend to darken because of friction and sunlight.

Prevention

To prevent age spots from occurring and freckles from multiplying and darkening, stay out of the sun! The more you worship the sun, the more lovely brown spots your skin will probably sport. If your knees and elbows tend to darken easily, avoid leaning on your elbows as much as possible and avoid floor exercises that call for you to be on your knees.

Treatments for Hyperpigmentation

When I hit my early thirties, I suddenly developed an on-again/off-again case of very mild adult acne that left small, brownish purple spots on my cheeks and jawline after the pimples had healed. Unlike my teenage pimples that healed without a trace, these spots remained visible for approximately 6 weeks before fading. I found this quite aggravating and resorted to wearing makeup to cover them, until I found an at-home treatment that works like a charm. I still use it to keep my skin smooth and skin tone even.

Twice a week I use an unripened green papaya enzyme mask that softens and exfoliates. It's gentle enough to be used around my eyes, too. Two to three times a week, before I go to bed, I apply a mild glycolic acid gel to my just-cleansed skin, then follow with a light moisturizer if I need one. Both the mask and the gel are completely natural and can be purchased from most natural products suppliers. You can use this combination of products wherever your skin needs to be lightened and the texture refined. I always wear a sunscreen to prevent damaging and darkening of my newly exfoliated skin.

Consulting the Experts

See an Esthetician If: For bit more aggressive approach to lightening your skin, your esthetician has access to products such as alpha-hydroxy acid peels, enzyme peels, glycolic acids, and quality skin-lightening formulas that contain 1 or 2 percent hydroquinone (a depigmentation agent that suppresses melanin pigment formation within the upper layers of the skin). Many of her products have higher concentrations of natural acids and enzymes than those that are available to you over the counter and she is well educated in their proper use.

See a Dermatologist If: If your "spots" are a bit resistant to your home or esthetician's remedies, a dermatologist may prescribe topical agents such as retinoic acid (Retin-A) cream or alpha- and beta-hydroxy acids combined with prescription-strength hydroquinone. Dermatologists have had great success using these ingredients to even out patients' skin tone and give a smooth texture to the skin. Some people, though, are sensitive to hydroquinone and it should be used with caution.

If you have a brown spot or two that is changing color and/or size, please bring this to the attention of your doctor so that she can treat it accordingly.

LEMON CREAM SKIN LIGHTENER

Lemon juice acts as an alpha-hydroxy acid and bleach, potato acts as an enzyme, cucumber acts as a cooling agent, and yogurt contains lactic acid and also acts as a bleach.

> 2 tablespoons (30 ml) fresh lemon juice
> 1 small potato, peeled
> ½ small cucumber
> 1 tablespoon (15 ml) plain, organic, raw yogurt (if raw is unavailable, then make sure it is minimally processed with no fillers and contains live cultures)

To make: Using a blender or small food processor, blend all ingredients until a smooth, spreadable paste is formed. Press mixture through a strainer if consistency is a bit lumpy. If the mixture is stored in a tightly covered container it will keep in refrigerator for 24 hours.

To use: Pull your hair up off your face and neck. Lie down with a towel under your head and neck to catch drips as this recipe can get a bit messy. Apply puree to face, neck, and chest, and cover with a hot, damp towel. For ease of breathing, you may want to use 2 hot towels, one to be draped from the tip of your nose up over your forehead and the other from your upper lip, down over your neck and chest. Leave skin lightener on for 15–20 minutes. Rinse, and follow with moisturizer if necessary. May be used twice weekly.

During the treatment, if your skin tingles a little, that's okay, but if it really begins to sting, rinse the puree off immediately and apply aloe vera gel, lavender hydrosol spray, chilled German chamomile tea, or plenty of cool water.

Caution: Do not use on inflamed, sunburned, or sensitive skin.

Yield: 1–2 treatments

POISON IVY, OAK, AND SUMAC

The irritating poison trio — the menace of summer wood-lands! Many people come in contact with these plants when wandering through the woods. Depending upon the sensi-tivity of your skin and the amount of exposure, symptoms may take a few hours or as much as a few days to appear. Minor itching and burning along with a red, slightly raised rash are the first signs, followed by the formation of small blisters that eventually rupture and form a crust.

Causes

The itchiness and irritation is caused by *urushiol,* the extremely irritating oily resin common to all three plants. Some people are immune to its effects, while others have severe reactions. Typically, severe reactions occur only if the plant resin comes in contact with your eyes, throat, feet, fin-gers, or groin, or if you constantly scratch the irritation.

Run-ins with poison ivy, oak, and sumac usually occur only during the warmer months, but that's not to say that you're completely safe during the winter, as my husband, Bill, found out. He owns a tree removal service and must occasionally climb a tree if it can't be reached with his bucket truck. One November, he was high in a large pine tree untan-gling a huge vine from its upper limbs when it occurred to him that the little white berries stemming from the vine trunk belonged to poison ivy. He had to handle that thick vine all day, but two days later he suffered only from a minor rash. I, on the other hand, was unlucky enough to load the washing

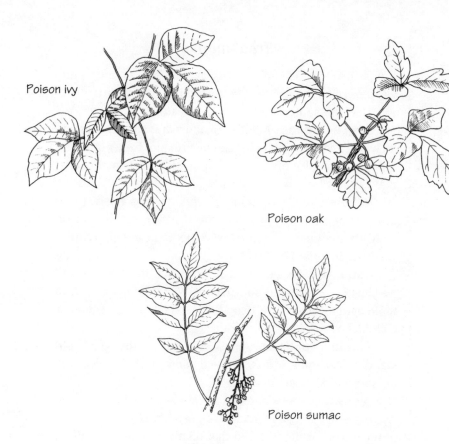

Poison ivy

Poison oak

Poison sumac

machine that evening. I must have gotten exposed to the sap from his clothes and developed a large, itchy, oozing patch of poison ivy on my thigh that lasted for 6 weeks! I am so much more sensitive to the irritating sap than he is.

Prevention

Learn to identify the plants in both summer and winter. An ounce of prevention is definitely worth a pound of cure! If you know you're going to be walking through areas where these plants are common, protect yourself by wearing long sleeves, pants, and boots. If you do have a run-in with any of them, wash your clothing in hot water immediately after arriving home — while wearing gloves — so it doesn't come in contact with other clothes and spread the poisonous agent.

Treatments

If possible, stay as cool and dry as possible, as hot, humid weather seems to exacerbate the itching (and your irritability). Here are some simple at-home treatments:

Soap and water. A hot soap and water shower immediately after contact will help remove urushiol from your skin. The hot water also often brings dramatic symptomatic relief that can last for hours.

Rubbing alcohol. Rubbing alcohol acts as a solvent for urushiol and can be applied to the affected area(s) immediately after coming in contact with the plant to help remove the irritating plant oil.

Oatmeal bath. For most minor reactions, doctors and herbalists recommend soaking for 20 to 30 minutes in a tepid bath to which ½ to 1 cup (125–250 ml) finely ground or colloidal oatmeal has been added.

Anti-itch potions. Aloe vera gel or the good old standby, calamine lotion, applied topically helps heal the blisters and alleviate itching.

Diet supplements. As an adult, I am now highly sensitive to these plants and must take precautions when walking in the woods or fields. I find that taking 500 to 1,000 mg of vitamin C helps prevent infection and the spread of the rash. The blisters seems to dry up faster, too!

CAUTION

If your case of poison plant rash develops in your eyes, throat, or groin region, or if it becomes raw, severely blistered, or possibly infected, consult with your doctor immediately. Aside from being uncomfortable, a bad rash can be a threat to your health.

Consulting the Experts

See an Esthetician If: I wouldn't advise seeing an esthetician when afflicted with this type of dermatitis. Steam, massage, or any type of touching will only lead to more itching, making the urge to scratch unbearable.

See a Dermatologist If: If the itching is driving you absolutely crazy and home treatments aren't bringing any relief, see your doctor. He or she can prescribe topical or oral cortisone to relieve the itching and aid in healing. Children, in particular, may need these aids, as they have a tendency to scratch themselves raw.

PSORIASIS

Symptoms of this disease are raised, pinkish red, thick patches of skin, often covered with dry silvery gray scales, appearing on any part of the body, particularly the scalp, knees, elbows, fingernails, and lower back. As the top layer flakes off smaller red areas beneath are exposed, which then begin to grow, frequently becoming larger, thicker plaques or disc-shaped lesions. Psoriatic patches can itch, burn, or sting, depending on the severity of the disease. The disease generally develops slowly, typically followed by unexplained remissions and recurrences.

The symptoms can vary in severity from very mild, where the person doesn't realize they actually have the disease, to extremely debilitating psoriasis. As reported by the American Academy of Dermatology, "The most severe cases of psoriasis destroy the skin's protective functions, allowing the skin to lose fluids and nutrients; losing control of body

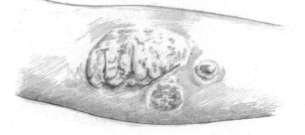

The elbow is one of the most common sites for the thick, scaly patches of skin that characterize psoriasis.

temperature; making patients susceptible to infection; and possibly causing death." The National Psoriasis Foundation estimates that four hundred people die from psoriasis-related causes each year.

A small percentage of psoriasis suffers are afflicted with arthritis. Sometimes the arthritis symptoms improve as the patient's skin condition improves.

Causes of Psoriasis

Psoriasis gets its name from the Greek word for "itch." It is not contagious and tends to be hereditary. The disease is caused by abnormal skin cell production. Normal skin cells mature every 28 to 35 days, depending on age, and are sloughed off unnoticed. When skin is affected by psoriasis, skin cells mature in 3 to 4 days, causing them to pile up and resulting in thick skin plaques. Their red appearance is due to the rich blood supply feeding the rapidly multiplying new skin cells.

There are several biochemical reactions that prompt this abnormal skin cell growth. They can be triggered by injury to the skin, some types of infection, a drug reaction, physical or emotional stress, or a surgical incision. Many herbalists suggest that it's a toxic liver or anxiety that causes psoriasis.

Prevention

If your parents suffered from psoriasis, chances are likely that you will too. But you can take measures to help prevent the disease from progressing. Eat a diet that is high in vitamins A, B, C, D, and E, zinc, and onions and garlic for their sulfur content. Supplements such as evening primrose oil or borage oil and supplement forms of the vitamins and minerals mentioned may be a prudent measure.

My skin care mentor, licensed esthetician Lozetta DeAngelo, believes that psoriasis is a stress-induced disease and suggests using stress reduction methods such as hypnosis, exercise, deep breathing, and yoga. She also says that due to today's agribusiness practices, our foods are not what they used to be nutritionally, thus our bodies suffer from a lack of vital nutrients and our skin reflects this deficiency.

Treatments for Psoriasis

Sunshine. The sun greatly aids in the healing of psoriasis lesions, but exposure to the sun can lead to premature aging, age spots, leathery skin, and possibly skin cancer. A few minutes spent in the sun in the morning and evening may prove beneficial, with minimal side effects, or you can apply sunscreen to all areas of your body except those affected by psoriasis and stay outside a bit longer.

CALENDULA OIL

This calendula-infused oil makes a soothing, gentle treatment for the itchy, sometimes painful symptoms of psoriasis, eczema, and even everyday rashes. It also makes a wonderful bath and massage oil.

> 2 cups (500 ml) dried calendula flowers (or 3 cups [750 ml] freshly wilted flowers — see page 145)
> 1 quart (1,000 ml) extra-virgin olive oil
> 1 tablespoon (15 ml) vitamin E oil

To make:
1. Pour the olive oil into a slow cooker or large saucepan and warm over the lowest possible heat setting. You want the oil to be just nicely warm, or about 125°F (50°C) — don't let it simmer. Add the flowers and stir to coat all the petals. Leave over heat for 12–24 hours, uncovered, stirring every few hours.
2. Strain the mixture through a mesh strainer lined with panty hose, catching the herbal oil in a bowl placed below. Press the remaining oil out of the flowers. (You can compost the spent flowers in your garden.)
3. Mix the vitamin E oil into the herbal oil. Store the oil in the refrigerator and use within 6 months.
To use: Rub right into any itchy, painful, dry spots; add a couple of tablespoons (30 ml) to a warm bath; use as a massage oil for normal-to-dry skin; or add to massage and facial oils as a soothing, moisturizing agent.
Yield: Approximately 1 quart (1 liter)

Diet. If self-treatment does not produce results, then a nutritionally oriented physician should be your second choice to get to the root of the cause of your suffering.

Calendula oil. Oil infused with calendula offers anti-inflammatory properties and can give both pain and itch relief for psoriatic lesions. It is a soothing, moisturizing, gentle preparation that can be used every day as necessary.

Treating Psoriasis: Tips from Stephan Brown, Herbalist

Stephan Brown, an herbalist friend and owner of The Great Cape Cod Herb, Spice & Tea Company, has seen many of his clients get dramatic relief from their psoriasis symptoms by consistently using his herbal Skin Ailment Assailment tea (page 142) together with his Comfrey/Calendula Healing Salve formula (page 144). He has kindly let me share his thoughts and his recipes with you. Should you want to purchase them ready-made, just give him a call and he'll gladly send you a fresh batch or two. Following is his advice and recipes.

A POEM FOR THE SKIN

Conditions of the skin may begin within
From fatty foods — (g)astronomical sin!
From foods that we eat that create body heat —
Like meat and wheat and far-too-sweet treats.

The fact of the matter (and the "why" of this chatter)
Is that what we INgest doesn't always DIgest
As well as it should, and so fouls the blood,
Thus breaking the skin from the shin to the chin!

The herbs in this blend may help make amends
For showing your liver disdain;
For they'll un-mud the blood, do their job with a nod
And deign to attain silky skin once again.

Calendula flow'r helps soothe itchy skin
And it's antibacterial to boot —
Burdock's for the liver, and cleansing the lymph —
The part that we use is the root.

And please do retain the tenacious Plantain
In the troops of your healing campaign;
For it takes out the zing
Of a bite, bruise, or sting
Of such tough conditions acute!

So when chemical drugs prove inefficacious,
Be sagacious in choosing these plants quite herbaceous;
That help bring a healing so gentle and gracious
With problems vexatious, epidermal, and sebaceous.

Problems of the skin must, of course, be treated systemically as well as topically. Many, such as eczema, psoriasis, and rashes, are the result of the body's accumulation of toxins: both endo-toxins (coming from within), which result from the natural processes of metabolism; and exo-toxins (coming from without), which come from the air we breathe, the food we ingest (including pesticides!), or in through the skin itself.

If the internal organs of elimination (lungs, liver, kidneys, and bowel) are unable to successfully deal with the toxic load, the body tries to push these wastes out through the skin — thus those unpleasant itches, rashes, and "breakout" conditions.

The herbs in the Skin Ailment Assailment formula (page 142) strengthen, nourish, energize, and soothe the organs of elimination so that these organs are better able to do their job of cleansing the body. When taking this remedy, it is usually a good sign if you feel worse before you feel better, for it indicates that the toxins are moving out of the liver and fatty tissue and into the bloodstream for eventual elimination through the kidneys.

A topical application of the Comfrey/Calendula Healing Salve (page 144) usually brings temporary relief, while the herbs taken internally, as either a tea or tincture, do their wonderful work of reestablishing internal homeostasis.

Do not ignore that diet is dramatically important in maintaining optimal health, including the health of the skin. Eat few fats and refined sugars and much "green leafies" and other vegetables. Make it a habit to eat like a rabbit!

Here are my formulas. May they bring you comfort and healing. Thanks for listening.

SKIN AILMENT ASSAILMENT TEA

All herbs in this formula are in dried form. It can be prepared as either a tea or a tincture.

- 4 parts burdock root
- 2 parts sassafras root bark
- 2 parts dandelion root
- 1 part Oregon grape root
- 1 part cinnamon bark granules (optional in tincture recipe)
- 1 part calendula flowers
- 1 part oat flowering tops
- 1 part echinacea herb or root
- 1 part nettle leaf
- 1 part cleavers herb

To make: Mix all herbs in a large bowl. Store in a tin, plastic tub, zip-seal plastic bag in a dark, dry cabinet or drawer. Will keep for up to 1 year.

To prepare a tea: Put 8 tablespoons (120 ml) of the herb mixture in a pot with ½ gallon (2 liters) water. Bring to a low simmer (do not let it boil!) and cook, covered, for ½ hour. Turn off heat and let stand for at least 2 hours — all day would be fine. Pour the mixture into a widemouthed jar and refrigerate. Each batch will last for 3–4 days.

To use the tea: Strain off each cup as needed. If your condition is severe, you could try 3–4 cups of tea per day. If you experience discomfort as the body begins to release toxins, reduce the amount (or stop altogether) until you are reasonably comfortable again, then begin to slowly increase your daily intake. Do not expect dramatic results until you have been on this protocol for at least 3–4 weeks (some individuals may notice changes more readily).

Tea yield: ½ gallon (2 liters)

To prepare a tincture: Place 3 cups (750 ml) of the herb mixture in a widemouthed quart (liter) jar. Cover with vodka (100 proof is best), with a mixture of 50 percent pure grain alcohol and 50 percent distilled water, or with organic vinegar. The liquid should be about 1 inch (2.5 cm) above the level of the herbs. Cover tightly. Shake several times a day for at least 2 weeks, preferably 3–4 weeks. Finally, strain through a cheesecloth or press with a potato ricer. Strain again into a dark glass bottle. From this master bottle, you may decant into a 2- or 4-ounce (60- or 125-ml) dropper-top bottle for easy dosing. Be sure to label all bottles and keep them out of reach of children.

To use the tincture: Half a teaspoon, 3 times a day in water or juice may be a good starting dose for a 150-pound (68-kg) adult. Adjust the amount for your constitution and size. Decrease amount as you begin to see results.

Tincture yield: Approximately 2–3 cups (500–750 ml), depending on how finely chopped the herbs are

How Much Is a "Part"?

A part can refer to any amount. It can mean teaspoons, tablespoons, cups, quarts, gallons, and so on. You assign a meaning to it depending upon how much formula you want to make. Half of a part will be half of whatever increment you are using. For instance, if in this recipe you decided that part would mean "cups," you'd have a whole lot of skin tea formula. If you decided that it would mean "teaspoons," then you'd be making enough for approximately 15 cups of skin tea, as the recipe calls for a total of 15 parts of herbs and it usually requires 1 teaspoon of dried herb per cup of boiling water. Understand?

Comfrey/Calendula Healing Salve

Formulated for treatment of psoriasis, this salve is also useful as a cuticle conditioner and can be used to soften dry feet, knees, elbows, and hands. This salve can also be used to heal and fade the appearance of scars.

1 quart (1 l) extra-virgin olive oil

¾ cup (180 ml) dried comfrey leaves

¾ cup (180 ml) dried calendula flowers

¾ cup freshly wilted St.-John's-wort flowers

½ scant cup (125 ml) dried plantain leaves

1 teaspoon (5 ml) myrrh gum resin powder

1 tablespoon (15 ml) vitamin E oil

½ cup (125 ml) beeswax

To find the flowers: The St.-John's-wort flowers are most potent when fresh, so the flowers used in this recipe must be freshly picked. If you don't grow St.-John's-wort in your garden, you'll have to wildcraft some blossoms for this recipe. St.-John's-wort can be found blooming in poor soil just about everywhere. It grows in masses up to 3 feet (1 m) tall and has a cheery, bright, small yellow flowers. Check a local flower guide to help you properly identify the plant. To help keep wild-growing populations of St.-John's-wort thriving, harvest just what you need, and don't harvest the entirety of any one population — leave enough that the plants will be able to regenerate. Do not harvest flowers from areas where pesticides are used or from the pollutant-filled areas near highways.

To make:

1. Add the olive oil to a slow cooker or 3-quart (3-l) saucepan and warm over the lowest possible heat setting. You want the oil to become just nicely warm — do not let it simmer! Add all of the ingredients except the vitamin E and beeswax. Stir thoroughly to coat the herbs with the oil and leave the heat for 12–24 hours, uncovered, stirring occasionally.

2. Strain the herbs through a potato ricer or mesh strainer lined with panty hose into a fresh bowl. Press the herbs in the strainer to squeeze out all of the oil. If you notice lots of particulate matter in the bottom of the bowl, you may want to restrain the liquid, but it's not necessary. Discard the spent herbs in your compost or garden.

3. In a 2-quart (2-l) saucepan, melt the beeswax over very low heat, then add the herbal oil. Stir to blend thoroughly, then remove from heat. You should have a slightly warm, golden-greenish oily liquid.

4. Stir in the vitamin E, which acts as a preservative. This recipe makes a large amount of salve, so you may want to pour it into four 8-ounce (225-g) jars or eight 4-ounce (115-g) jars for easier storage. If refrigerated, the salve will last for approximately 1 year; if left at room temperature, it should be used within 6 months.

To use: Apply this salve as often as necessary to soothe, soften, and heal dry, crusty psoriatic patches.

Yield: Approximately 1 quart (1 liter)

Wilting Flowers

Some herbal treatments, such as the Comfrey/Calendula Healing Salve and Calendula Oil (on page 139), call for "freshly wilted" flowers. Fresh and wilt may seem a contradiction of terms, but there is a reason for it: A day of wilting allows a large proportion of the water that flowers contain to evaporate, maximizing the potency of the preparation they'll be used in.

To wilt freshly picked flowers, spread them onto an herb-drying screen or lay them on newspaper that is covered with a layer of paper towels. Keep the flowers in a place that gets plenty of air circulation but is out of the sun and away from dirt. After 24 hours, the flowers should be nicely wilted and a large proportion of the water they contain should have evaporated.

Consulting the Experts

See an Esthetician If: The assistance your esthetician can provide is palliative at best. She is your best source, other than your dermatologist, for efficient moisturizing creams to help keep your psoriasis patches soft and flexible, minimizing dryness, cracking, and bleeding.

See a Dermatologist If: If your psoriasis condition continues to worsen, despite self-help remedies and nutritional therapy, see your dermatologist. She or he can prescribe relatively safe topical treatments such as tar and cortisone creams for a mild to moderate case, or oral medications for a more severe case. Be aware that these drugs are not without serious side effects. In my opinion, as with any disease condition, it is always best to seek alternative therapies before resorting to potentially harmful drug treatment.

ROSACEA

Rosacea is a highly visible disease, and left untreated can result in an unsightly appearance. According to the Spring 1998 issue of the *Rosacea Review,* "Rosacea is estimated to affect more than thirteen million Americans, and typically strikes after age thirty as a redness on the cheeks, nose, chin or forehead that comes and goes. Left untreated, the redness becomes ruddier and more permanent. Tiny dilated blood vessels may become visible, and acne-like bumps and pimples often appear.

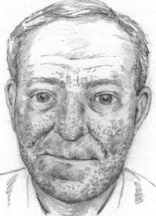

In advanced cases of rosacea, the redness is severe, tiny dilated blood vessels may become visible, acnelike bumps and pimples appear, and the nose may become bumpy and enlarged.

"In advanced cases, the nose may be come bumpy, red, and enlarged from excess tissue. In some individuals, rosacea also causes the eyes to become gritty and red as it increases in severity, potentially leading to vision loss."

SKINFORMATION

Those most likely to develop rosacea are adults, particularly women, between the ages of thirty and fifty who have fair skin, light eyes and hair, and sensitive skin. A condition called rhinophyma, found primarily in men, can develop in advanced stages of rosacea, in which the sebaceous glands become enlarged, lumpy, and unsightly, causing a bulbous nose and thickened, puffy cheeks. In severe cases the symptoms extend down to the jawline.

Remember W.C. Fields? He had a large, red, bulbous nose that most people mistakenly thought was due to alcoholism, but in actuality he had rosacea. However, alcohol *is* a trigger food that can greatly aggravate an existing rosacea condition.

Causes of Rosacea

There is no proven cause for rosacea. It is believed to be a vascular disorder with a constant cycle of inflammation, swelling, redness, blood vessel dilation, and acnelike symptoms.

Many estheticians I spoke to believe that rosacea is an adult skin's response to stress. I developed a mild case of rosacea during the winter of 1997. I thought it was adult acne, but my dermatologist told me that because of the constant redness, it was actually rosacea. I was undergoing lots of stress during the dry cold of a New England winter, and my skin responded unfavorably. A few months later, after my life had calmed down a bit, the symptoms went away and never returned.

Prevention

Rosacea is characterized by bouts of intense flare-ups followed by periods of blessed remission. There is no known preventive, but if you are predisposed to rosacea it is important to know that there are steps you can take to temper these flare-ups in mild to moderate cases. If you're suffering from a cold, the flu, or allergies, or going through menopause, you may be prone to a bout of rosacea, and there's not much you can do to prevent it. However, rosacea is triggered by many conditions and situations that you can avoid, including the following:

- Sunburn
- Temperature extremes
- Emotional stress
- Birth control pills
- Alcoholic drinks
- Intense exercise, especially weight lifting
- Hot, spicy drinks and foods; other foods such as caffeinated coffee or tea, dairy, wheat, citrus, eggplant, tomato, and salty condiments can also be triggers
- Acne medication, topical cortisone, or other medications that cause the blood vessels to dilate
- Harsh skin treatments and overzealous facial scrubbing using a facial exfoliant or washcloth, which can irritate an already reddened skin

Treatments for Rosacea

Rosacea is a chronic, progressive disease, and treatment should begin in the early stages before symptoms take a turn for the worse.

Cleansing. Avoid hot or cold water — use tepid water when washing and rinsing your skin. Avoid drying acne medications, which can further irritate inflamed skin. You need to use mild, fragrance-free, color-free, noncomedogenic products to keep skin smooth and hydrated. Add a few drops of German chamomile, lavender, or calendula essential oil to your products to calm redness and inflammation. Keep an aromatic hydrosol handy to prevent surface dryness.

Diet and supplements. Make sure that your diet contains more than ample amounts of vitamins A, B, C, D, and E; zinc; silicon; and evening primrose or borage oil. Include lots of fresh fruits, vegetables, and fiber.

Fluids. By all means, avoid constipation. You've got to keep those intestines clean and toxins movin' on out! So every day, drink plenty of water or healing herbal teas, such as Skin Tea.

SKIN TEA

~~~~~~

The Skin Tea I formulated," says Shatoiya de la Tour of Dry Creek Herb Farm and Learning Center, "is an all-purpose tea effective in many situations. I've had clients with rosacea find relief by drinking this tea and using it as a cold compress. I recommend it for burn victims, also. It is also a good support tea for any type of skin problem, such as acne, eczema, or psoriasis.

"Of course, you must realize that diet and lifestyle play a big part in the healing process. As an herbalist, I custom blend each tea or tincture based on a person's health history, family health history, and lifestyle."

    1½ parts dried nettle
     1 part dried calendula flowers
     1 part dried red clover flowers
    ½ part dried symphytum leaf (comfrey)
    ½ part dried lavender buds

To make: Bring 1 quart (1 liter) of water to a boil, remove from heat, and add 4–5 heaping teaspoons (20–25 ml) tea mixture. Cover and steep for 30 minutes to 1 hour. Strain.

To use: "I generally have my client make up a big pot and sip it all day from a big cup or thermos," says Shatoiya. She also recommends applying a cool compress of Skin Tea to inflamed, irritated areas of the face to help soothe and reduce any redness.

Yield: 1 quart (1 liter) of tea

DIETARY DO'S AND DON'TS

"In almost all skin problems, I've found that adding a daily or at least every other day supplement of 200–400 IUs of vitamin E and a good-quality evening primrose capsule to be beneficial," states herbalist Shatoiya de la Tour. "Especially with rosacea, but with other skin problems as well, cutting wheat and dairy out of the diet is essential. Do this strictly for at least three months and then you can add in some of these foods occasionally."

Consulting the Experts

See an Esthetician If: A skin suffering from rosacea symptoms has thriving bacteria colonies forming under the skin. Your esthetician can gently deep cleanse your skin, removing impurities. She can also apply a series of mild glycolic acid peels to help remove dead surface skin, which should gradually improve your overall appearance.

See a Dermatologist If: Rosacea is best treated in the early stages. Try to locate an herbal or nutritionally oriented doctor first, to try to balance your system and prevent progression of the disease. In moderate to severe cases, topical and oral antibacterial treatments may be prescribed by your doctor, but these are not without potentially harmful side effects.

SCARS AND KELOIDS

A scar forms as your skin repairs a wound caused by an accident, surgical procedure, disease, or severe sunburn. It is formed by the natural healing processes of your body. Scars can be raised or flat; long, short, or round; and flesh toned, pink, purple, or brown in color.

Causes

Some people are more likely than others to develop problem scars and scars that are resistant to fading. A scar's formation and appearance will depend on your health, age, skin type, skin color, and the particular conditions surrounding the initial trauma. The degree to which a scar develops greatly depends on the severity of the damage to the skin and the length of time it takes to heal. The longer the healing process and the more the skin is damaged, the increased likelihood of a noticeable scar.

A hypertrophic scar has scar tissue that is elevated above the surface of the skin and the tissue forms in direct proportion to the size of the wound. A keloid is similar to the hypertrophic scar, except that the scar tissue forms out of proportion to the amount of scar tissue normally required for repair and healing. In other words, it extends beyond the boundaries of the original wound site and into the surrounding skin. Black skin is prone to the development of keloids.

Prevention

If you don't want to risk getting a scar at some point in your life, then you need to live in a bubble. However, once you do have an injury, the best way to prevent the growth of scar tissue or at least minimize its growth is to begin proper care of the wound and treatment of the potential scar site at once and avoid further injury to the wound site.

SKINFORMATION

According to the American Academy of Dermatology, "A scar's visibility will depend on a number of factors, including its color, texture, depth, length, width, or direction. How the scar forms will also be affected by an individual's age and by its location on the body or face."

Treatments for Scars

Everyone's skin is unique and reacts differently to different products, so keep that in mind when self-treating scars. For assistance, your local pharmacist is a good person to consult about nonprescription topical scar treatments.

Older scars, raised scars, long surgical scars, or those that develop and deepen over time, such as acne and chickenpox scars, can be difficult or impossible to treat with a home remedy and should be addressed by a dermatologist if they cause any discomfort.

Vitamin E oil. Vitamin E oil has been used successfully by many people to help soften and fade all types of scars. Pierce several vitamin E gel capsules and spread the contents over the affected area.

Herbal ointments and salves. Ointments and salves containing St.-John's-wort, calendula, and comfrey work well to prevent the formation of scars as well as heal and fade existing scars. Stephan Brown's formula for Calendula/Comfrey Healing Salve (on page 144) is a good example.

Wild Rose Oil. My friend and fellow herbalist, Julie Bailey, owner of Mountain Rose Herbs, has kindly agreed to share her herbal oil recipe with you. It's easy to make and smells delightful, too! If you'd rather purchase a bottle, it is available in her retail catalog (see resources).

Consulting the Experts

See an Esthetician If: If you have minor acne scarring or uneven skin tone, your esthetician can administer a series of glycolic acid peels, to gradually minimize your scars and even out your skin tone. She can also provide you with collagen fiber strips that work wonderfully for softening the appearance of new scars.

See a Dermatologist If: To alter the appearance of moderate to severe scars, visiting a dermatologist is your best bet. He can provide the medical technique best suited to your particular type of scar. These techniques can include deep chemical peels, surgical scar revision, punch grafts, cryosurgery, dermabrasion, temporary collagen injections, and laser surgery.

WILD ROSE OIL

This exquisite blend is an all-purpose facial and body oil that is rejuvenating and restoring. It produces great results on skin damaged by acne, scars, and sun, and is also beneficial for mature, and dry skin. It contains rosehip seed oil, which is highly regenerative to skin tissue.

20 drops lavender (Lavandula angustifolia) essential oil
10 drops carrot seed essential oil
15 drops everlasting essential oil
6 tablespoons (90 ml) wild rosehip seed oil
2 tablespoons (30 ml) calendula oil (see page 139 for recipe)
2 tablespoons (30 ml) jojoba oil (organic, if possible)
1 teaspoon (5 ml) vitamin E oil (food grade, wheatgerm oil base)

To make:
1. Combine the essential oils, lavender, carrot seed, and everlasting, in a small bottle and allow to sit for at least 2 hours. I suggest using a labeled amber glass bottle, stored away from children and pets.
2. Combine the wild rosehip seed, calendula, and jojoba oils in an glass bottle. Add the essential oil blend and the vitamin E oil, and shake thoroughly.
Note: It is important to blend the essential oils and the base oils well. The jojoba oil is actually a liquid wax that will tend to separate if not blended completely. The oil will keep for up to 1 year if stored in a dark, cool cabinet.
To use: Apply a dab of oil onto scar tissue twice daily and gently massage in. Use consistently for several months until you are pleased with the results.
Yield: Approximately 5 ounces (150 ml)

SHAVING IRRITATIONS

Men share many of the same skin care concerns as women — oiliness, blackheads, pimples, dryness, flaking, and wrinkles — but in addition, they also have their own unique set of problems. What do just about all men have in common? They shave their faces and irritation from shaving and lack of proper follow-up care often leads to skin complaints. Nicks, cuts, scrapes, razorburn, and bleeding skin — improper shaving can leave a man's face feeling like raw meat. Add the problem of ingrown hairs and you've got the potential for developing an unattractive infection.

Causes

The act of shaving is not itself harmful to the skin. On the contrary, it thoroughly exfoliates the face and neck and reveals smooth, new skin. Men who shave their faces, just as people who apply exfoliating masks and scrubs, are working to improve the texture of their skin.

Pseudofolliculitis is a condition that affects men with stiff, heavy beards, particularly adult black males. Instead of emerging from the hair follicle, newly growing hair tips stay subsurface and enter the surrounding skin, inducing inflammation surrounding the follicle. The condition appears as inflamed, red bumps and can easily be mistaken for acne. The condition will persist as long as the man continues to shave, possibly leaving scars.

To remedy the situation, estheticians recommend following a warm shower or hot towel application with a facial scrub 2 to 3 times a week to help loosen imbedded hairs and remove surface buildup of dead skin. Alternatively, you could always grow a beard and the condition will take care of itself.

Pseudofolliculitis could be mistaken for acne, but it's actually infected hair follicles caused by shaving.

Professional Shaving Tips

I consulted a local barber on how to do a professional and comfortable shave. The primary business for most barbers is giving haircuts, but there are a few men who still enjoy a good shave, I was told.

First, the barber applies a warm, damp towel to the face and neck for a couple of minutes to soften the beard and then slathers on a conditioning cream (not soap). Next he uses a sharp straight razor to slowly and cleanly cut the beard. He cleans up with a warm towel, then applies a conditioning aftershave with minimal alcohol content. Notice that I said sharp razor. A dull razor results in nicks, cuts, and abrasions because the blade doesn't glide smoothly across the skin, thus making you apply more pressure to get the job done.

What do most men slap on their skin after a shave? Generally an alcohol-based aftershave lotion. Granted, the immediate effect is cooling and bracing to the skin, but to many, it also stings a bit, especially if you're bleeding or have sensitive skin. As the aftershave dries and the alcohol evaporates from the skin's surface, the skin is left in a dehydrated state. This is why you see many men, particularly in early spring, fall, and winter, with dry skin and premature wrinkling around their eyes.

Follow these shaving tips for smoother, brighter skin:

- Always soften your beard and hydrate your skin prior to shaving. This makes cutting the beard hairs much easier and softens embedded sebum.
- Always apply a conditioning shaving cream to help your razor glide across your skin.
- Use a sharp razor at all times, changing the blade at least once a week.
- Take your time — a rush job looks and feels terrible. No need to face the world with bloody battle scars.
- Use a conditioning aftershave balm and always follow with moisturizer unless you have very oily skin.
- If you have pimples or acne, be extra careful not to shave the pimples and cause further inflammation. An electric razor may be less irritating.

Treatments

To avoid facial irritation resulting from shaving, men need to follow a simple, basic skin care routine. Don't worry, I'm not going to recommend anything complicated requiring scads of potions and lotions that you have to carry to work with you for midday maintenance. What I'm suggesting here are simple, easy-to-follow steps to ensure clear, supple, appealing skin.

If you're like most men, you like to shower, shave, and go, no time to fuss over appearances. But, if you'd just take a little more time to care for your skin properly, I'd be willing to bet that your spouse or partner may actually find you more attractive.

Step 1: Cleansing. If you wish to continue using soap to wash your face and for shaving preparation, at least purchase either a goat milk or superfatted soap to help counteract the resulting dryness. Preferably, choose an inexpensive, gentle cleansing lotion available from the health food store or drugstore. Nothing fancy — just a basic nondrying formula.

Step 2: Aftershave. For your aftershave balm — to tighten skin as well as condition — try my Spicy Aftershave (on page 157). If you're not interested in making your skin care wares, try using plain witch hazel, available from the drugstore. It has a low alcohol content.

Step 3: Moisturizing. Use a moisturizer designed for your skin type. It would be best to use a moisturizing sunscreen every day, 365 days a year, to protect and hydrate and to help prevent skin cancer, age spots, and premature wrinkling.

Step 4: Once a week. Apply a clay-based facial scrub-mask combo to cleanse pores and refine texture (such as the Mountain Rose Facial Scrub on page 168), or purchase a ready-made product from a health food store or through mail order (see resources). Concentrate on the nose and forehead where shaving doesn't take place and blackheads tend to accumulate.

Spicy Aftershave

2 cups (500 ml) witch hazel (available in drugstores)

2 4" (10 cm) sprigs fresh rosemary

2 4" (10 cm) sprigs fresh mint of choice

2 cinnamon sticks

20 whole cloves

2 strips of fresh orange peel (organically grown, if possible), about 4" long and ½" wide

2 strips of fresh lemon peel (organically grown, if possible), about 4" long and ½" wide

1 teaspoon (5 ml) jojoba or almond oil

1 teaspoon (5 ml) vegetable glycerin

10 drops orange, lemon, or lime essential oil (omit these oils if you have sensitive skin)

To make: Place all ingredients in a 1-quart (1-liter) canning jar. Cover the top of the jar with plastic wrap, then screw on the lid (the plastic prevents the lid from rusting). Store in a dark place for 2 weeks, shaking daily. Strain into a decorative bottle with either a spray top or plastic cap. If you wish, you may put a fresh cinnamon stick in the bottle to enhance its esthetics. There's no need to refrigerate this formula, but you should use it within 6 months.

To use: Shake before each use. Apply generously after shaving; follow with the appropriate moisturizer for your skin type.

Yield: 2 cups (500 ml)

Treatments for Razorburn

Do you suffer from itchy, burning, or red, rashy skin immediately after shaving your legs, bikini line, or underarms? Razorburn affects many women, especially those with sensitive or fair skin. To prevent razorburn, always use an ultra-sharp razor blade, and change blades after every third or fourth shave. To soothe the irritation and reduce inflammation, follow these tips after shaving:

◆ For legs, apply a cold body lotion. (Store the lotion in the refrigerator — it's super-refreshing in the summer!)

◆ Spray irritated areas with a chilled bottle of German chamomile or lavender hydrosol, or aloe vera juice.

◆ Combine ½ cup (125 ml) witch hazel with 10 drops of calendula or lavender essential oil in a spray bottle, and spritz on irritated areas as needed. For maximum potency, use within 6 months and shake well before each use.

Consulting the Experts

See an Esthetician If: If you have a case of pseudofolliculitis, a visit to a good esthetician can dramatically improve the situation.

See a Dermatologist If: A severe case of pseudofolliculitis may require a doctor's visit, but usually an esthetician can take care of this problem.

SUNBURN

We've all had a sunburn at least one time in our lives. A first-degree sunburn is the most common. First you burn, turn red, tender, and sting, then in a few days your skin begins to peel, and then it returns to normal, or so it seems. Maybe you get a tan instead of peeling. That's how my skin reacted as a child, but now, at thirty-six, I'm beginning to get age spots. *C'est la vie!*

A second degree sunburn is a severe burn that results in chills, blisters, a painful headache, and occasionally fever. Your skin stings and itches and you basically feel miserable. After-effects of such trauma can be scarring and changes in the texture of your skin.

SKINFORMATION

According to Arthur K. Balin, M.D., Ph.D., and Loretta Pratt Balin, M.D., authors of *The Life of the Skin: What It Hides, What It Reveals, and How It Communicates,* "Eventually a sunburn or suntan recedes, perhaps giving the impression that any damage that was done is gone forever. But skin, like film, is capable of registering light and storing it in its genetic memory, the DNA. With time as the developer, the memory of that light may emerge many years later, revealing its stored imprint in the form of wrinkles, liver spots, and other sun damage. When DNA is damaged by UV or some other agent, it may correct itself by means of one of several cellular mechanisms. The genetic damage may be repaired before it is carried on any further, like a run in a stocking that is stopped before it extends the whole length of the leg. However, if none of these repair pathways are activated, the future of the affected cells is unpredictable. A mutation in only one cell is all that is required to start a cancer."

Causes of Sunburn

Ultraviolet light from the sun is the villain, and it consists of three subgroups: UVA, UVB, and UVC.

UVA, according to the American Cancer Society, "can be up to one thousand times more intense than UVB and can penetrate the skin to cause damage to underlying tissue. UVA is considered to be the primary cause of long-term skin damage from the sun (photoaging). In response to UVB and UVA exposure, existing melanocytes (your skin's pigment cells) move closer to the skin's surface and more melanocytes are produced. The result is your body's own way of protecting you — a tan." UVA also promotes dryness, wrinkles, uneven skin tone, and leathery skin. While UVB rays are strongest between the hours of 10:00 A.M. and 2:00 P.M., UVA radiation affects you from dawn to dusk, creating long-term damage that accelerates the skin's aging process and encourages the breakdown of collagen. UVA rays also cause an increased risk of skin cancer.

UVB light causes the most sunburns. Most sunscreens will effectively block up to 94 to 97 percent of UVB rays, but not UVA rays.

UVC is a type of ultraviolet light that's not heard about very often. It is almost completely absorbed by the ozone layer of our atmosphere, is potentially the most carcinogenic of the UV subgroups, and is deadly to animal and plant life. Additionally, for you tanning-bed lovers out there, UVC is also created by artificial light. I don't care what the nice person behind the counter at the tanning salon tells you when you fork over your membership money — tanning beds are not safe!

Prevention

Common sense and a daily dose of sunscreen is your best bet for preventing sunburn, plain and simple. Make sure that the sunscreen you choose has a strength of at least SPF (sun protection factor) 15 and says somewhere on the label that it provides UVA and UVB Broad Spectrum Protection. Your sunscreen should also be greaseless, fragrance-free, comfortable under makeup, and water resistant or water-

TEACHING OUR CHILDREN ABOUT THE SUN

If you read the section on skin cancer (pages 89–96), you're aware of the dangers of overexposure to the sun. Children need to be educated and protected. Though it is recommended that all children wear hats, protective clothing, sunglasses, and play in the shade, most won't. So, what to do? At least 30 minutes before they go off to school or out to play, make it a practice to apply sunscreen to your children yourself, rather than letting them do it. This way they'll learn the appropriate amount to put on their skin and hopefully this daily routine will become a lifelong habit.

Remember the thick white stuff lifeguards used to put on their noses? That old standby, white zinc oxide cream, is still available, but is now also offered in colors kids love. It totally blocks the sun and kids like the shocking colors, so they don't mind wearing it!

proof for good staying power. It should also dry quickly. If you're going to be outside exercising, doing manual labor, swimming at the beach, or cutting the grass, make sure your sunscreen is waterproof and sweatproof, not just water resistant.

If you're sensitive to chemical sunscreens, my favorite natural sunscreens are the titanium dioxide–based products available on the market today. Titanium dioxide is a natural mineral that acts as a good physical block to UVA and UVB rays. Zinc oxide cream, that familiar white cream commonly used by children, lifeguards, and ski instructors on their most highly sensitive and exposed areas — such as on their noses, cheeks, and shoulders — also makes an effective physical barrier to the sun, if you don't mind greasy white stripes decorating your face and body.

Treatments for Sunburn

A sunburn will dehydrate your skin, make the collagen fibers less flexible, destroy the protective acid mantle, and leave you looking like a shedding reptile. It's essential to rehydrate your skin immediately following a burn to restore pH balance and soothe the tender, delicate, injured tissue.

For a first- or second-degree sunburn, you need to reduce the temperature of the skin by applying a cold, wet washcloth to the affected area(s) or by taking a cool bath or shower. Pat your skin dry, then generously spray on some Aloe After-Sun Relief Spray. Follow up with a good moisturizer, preferably one with German chamomile essential oil, to help reduce inflammation and restore pliability to your dried-out skin. Always pat on your moisturizer — rubbing or massaging sunburned skin will simply add insult to injury.

ALOE AFTER-SUN RELIEF SPRAY

1 cup (250 ml) store-bought aloe vera juice (not gel)
40 drops lavender essential oil
20 drops calendula essential oil
20 drops carrot seed essential oil
5 drops peppermint or rosemary, chemotype verbenon essential oil (optional, for cooling effect)

To make: Place all ingredients in an 8-ounce (250 ml) dark glass spray bottle and shake well. This formula can be stored in the refrigerator for up to 6 months.
To use: Spray on sensitive burned skin as often as necessary to help hydrate and soothe, and prevent infection and scarring.
Yield: 1 cup (250 ml)

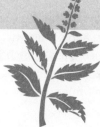

Sunburn Relief for Children

Inevitably, children will get sunburned at some point in their young lives, so here is a hydrating herbal spray to help relieve the pain of sunburn. This formula is exceptionally mild yet effective and can be used even on infants.

¼ cup (60 ml) distilled water
¼ cup (60 ml) store-bought aloe vera juice (not the gel)
5 drops lavender, calendula, or German chamomile essential oil

To make: Combine ingredients in a 4-ounce (115-ml) spray bottle. This formula can be stored in refrigerator for 4–6 months.

To use: Shake well before each use and spray directly onto sunburned skin as often as necessary to ease pain and help prevent peeling. Do not spray directly into eyes.

Yield: ½ cup (125 ml)

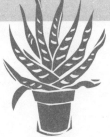

Consulting the Experts

See an Esthetician If: If summer sun or a midwinter vacation to the tropics has left your complexion parched, flaky, and unevenly toned, visit your esthetician for a skin-plumping, rehydrating, gently exfoliating facial and/or body treatment.

See a Dermatologist If: If you have a severe sunburn over a large portion of your body and develop chills, fever, or a bad headache, see your doctor immediately or pay a visit to the emergency room. A second-degree sunburn can be extremely painful and cause you to become very ill.

WRINKLES

Life is an ongoing adventure for your skin, a journey of days and nights filled with sun, wind, temperature extremes, late nights, smoke and pollution, stress, and skin care neglect. Wrinkles aren't a "problem" per se, but a natural evolution of life's toll on your features. Although you can't prevent wrinkles, you can learn to slow the hands of time and retain your youthful glow for years to come with gentle, natural care and maintenance procedures. Chapter 7 addresses the specifics of care and treatment for each generation.

CHAPTER 7
Skin Challenges to Expect from Your Twenties through Your Seventies

▼▼▼

About face . . . forward march — gracefully! This chapter is about how to attain and maintain "skin wellness" throughout your lifetime. It's also about what skin challenges or changes to expect, and what to do about them. I'll show you how to fortify your skin and promote its optimal health and good looks so you can be the best you possible, at any age!

What's practically poreless and a flawless picture of plump perfection? A baby's skin! From the moment we're born, the genetic clock starts ticking and doesn't stop until we die. Aging is inevitable, unfortunately. However, many of the signs of "aging" are self-inflicted, due to neglect or excessive exposure to environmental factors such as sun, wind, cold, heat, or pollution. Poor dental health, sagging, wrinkled skin, hyperpigmentation, bad posture, obesity, flabby muscles, and a dry, dull, lifeless complexion are signs of deterioration that you can control to a large degree.

I, like many people, am choosing to accept the aging process with dignity and grace. But I do want to retain and maintain my youthfulness as long as I can. Instead of fighting this natural process every step of the way and cursing my skin changes, I've educated myself and learned that through diet, exercise, stress relief, and regular skin care procedures, I can look forward to a lifetime of radiant skin.

CHRONOLOGICAL AGING VERSUS PHOTOAGING

"Time changes things." An old adage, but one that rings true. Like a fine wine, you can get better with age if you take care of yourself.

There are two types of aging: chronological aging and photoaging or environmental aging. Chronological aging of the skin occurs from preprogrammed genetic factors, and there is nothing you can do about it. Your skin, its particular characteristics, and any associated aging idiosyncrasies that come along with it are an inherited gift from your mother and father.

However, most visible signs of aging, from age spots to wrinkles to a leathery texture, are not the result of the years you've lived, but rather a result of the "light" years you've received — photoaging. In other words, photoaging is the result of years of unprotected, chronic sun exposure superimposed on the chronological aging process. Other environmental factors and lifestyle habits contribute to this process as well.

In actuality, depending on the genes you were dealt, your state of health, and the level of care given your skin, your skin at age thirty-five can be of almost the same quality at age fifty. You can, in all reality, maintain that youthful glow well beyond the average time limit. Or the reverse can occur. An overstressed, out of shape, unhealthy man or woman of thirty-five can look older than a fifty year old who takes care of him or herself.

The never-ending search for the fountain of youth continues — will we ever find our Shangri-La, our Utopia, where skin has nary a wrinkle, crease, discolored spot, or blemish? Where everyone is physically beautiful and never shows signs of old age? That's doubtful, but science will keep trying.

I feel that beauty is comprised of your personality, your poise, and your smile — including those laugh lines! You alone are responsible for your inner glow and outer radiance and should embrace your advancing years. You can choose to age naturally and gracefully, welcoming your skin's changes, or you can neglect yourself, do nothing, and age prematurely. Remember, it's not the passing of the years that ages you, but how you care or fail to care for yourself. No one knows when their first line or next wrinkle will appear, but you should become aware of how to deal with the skin challenges ahead and be armed with knowledge to combat or soften the signs of aging.

YOUR YOUTHFUL TWENTIES

Ah, your twenties. Your skin is in its prime — beautiful, glowing radiance that's evenly toned and smooth. One of the joys of youth! Skin at this age is strong and resilient, with good elasticity and a firm, smooth appearance. It's usually problem free.

Gentle Treatments for a Lifelong Healthy Complexion

You may still be plagued with T-zone oiliness, acne, and blemishes if you experienced these afflictions during your teenage years, but don't continue to treat these problems with the same harsh products you probably used in years past. Kinder, gentler products are more beneficial now and won't leave the surface of your skin dehydrated.

The late twenties may present signs of early dryness and the beginning signs of sun damage if you roasted yourself as a child: treat these problems accordingly. To foster a lifetime of healthy, supple skin, you need to begin to combat signs of aging. So if you ignored your skin in your younger years, by all means start now to lay a good foundation for the years ahead.

Julie Bailey of Mountain Rose Herbs sells the Mountain Rose facial scrub recipe on page 168 through her mail-order catalog. It's simple to make and doubles as a gentle exfoliating mask if allowed to dry on your skin for 15 to 30 minutes. With repeated use, it will remove deep-seated impurities, leaving your skin soft, supple, and glowing.

Skin Care Specifics for the Twenties

◆ Use sun protection daily with an SPF of at least 15.

◆ Wash gently — avoid overzealous scrubbing and harsh cleansers.

◆ Cleanse thoroughly. Rinse, rinse, and rinse to remove excess cleanser and debris that could clog pores.

◆ Use a mild moisturizer formulated for your skin type at all times (or a sunscreen/moisturizer combination) to keep skin hydrated and prevent premature crinkling around the lips and eyes.

◆ See your dermatologist if you have acne and it is not responding to home treatments. Avoid picking skin to prevent further inflammation and scarring.

◆ Choose noncomedogenic makeup and skin care products to prevent clogging of pores.

◆ Wash makeup applicators approximately once a week and keep them clean.

◆ Quit smoking and drinking alcohol and caffeinated drinks. These bad habits only serve to remove nutrients and moisture from the body.

◆ Keep your stress under control.

MOUNTAIN ROSE FACIAL SCRUB

This formula, created by Julie Bailey of Mountain Rose Herbs, is beneficial for oilier skins with mild acne, or those certain times of the month when a woman's skin may be oilier. It can be used on the legs, arms, and chest as well as the face and makes an excellent spot-treatment mask for specific oily areas.

4 drops juniper berry essential oil

3 drops lavender angustifolia essential oil

1 drop thyme or tea tree essential oil

2 tablespoons (30 ml) almond meal (see page 57; about 25 medium fresh, raw almonds)

4 tablespoons (60 ml) French green clay

2 tablespoons (30 ml) oat bran or finely ground oatmeal

½ tablespoon (8 ml) comfrey root powder

To make:

1. Combine essential oils in a small bottle and allow to sit for a minimum of 2 hours.

2. Use a whisk to press through a sieve first the almond meal, then the clay. Repeat with the oat bran and comfrey root powder. Stir/whisk well.

3. Add the essential oil blend to the bowl a little at a time, whisking thoroughly after each addition. Cover the bowl with a clean, dry cloth or other dry cover, and allow scrub to sit 4–8 hours.

4. Whisk again, then scoop the mixture into a jar with an airtight lid. Use within 1 month, or store in the refrigerator for up to 3 months.

To use: Scoop 1 teaspoon to 1 tablespoon (5–15 ml) into the palm of your hand. Add sufficient water or herbal tea (peppermint, yarrow, or sage are good choices) to make a paste. Cleanse your face and throat using small, circular motions.

To use as a facial mask: This scrub can also be left on as a facial mask by adding enough of any of the following liquids to make a paste:

- ◆ **Astringent** — Peppermint, yarrow, or sage tea
- ◆ **Calming** — German chamomile or lavender hydrosol
- ◆ **Nourishing** — Yogurt
- ◆ **Softening** — Avocado
- ◆ **Refreshing** — Mango
- ◆ **Moisturizing** — Honey
- ◆ Or a combination of any of the above!

Rinse with warm, then cool water. For facial use a twice-weekly treatment as a mask or scrub is sufficient for all skin types. As a body scrub, one or two treatments a week are sufficient.

Contraindication: Do not use this formula if you suffer from severe acne or couperose skin, as it could further aggravate the condition.

Yield: Approximately 8–16 treatments

THE CHANGEABLE THIRTIES

"Ye reap what ye sow." Thus begins the decade where your past skin sins will come back to haunt you. Your days of fun in the sun will become visible as an outcropping of fine lines and creases materializes around your eyes and lips and age spots emerge where once there was uniformly colored skin. Remember, your skin reflects accumulated environmental damage. I know a woman who grew up on the Florida beaches. Her dark, rich, teenage tan was the envy of all her friends. She is only six years older than I am, but now looks at least twice that!

Some women are beginning their childbearing years during this decade; others are ending theirs. Hormonal swings from birth control pills, stress, or pregnancy can wreak havoc on an otherwise normal skin. Adult acne can flare up even if you never had it in your youth. It will usually rear its ugly head on the lower cheeks and jawline, but can occur anywhere on the face. See chapter 6 for this specific skin care concern.

Oil production begins to decrease as you age, which can be a boon for those with oily skin, but a curse for those with normal-to-dry skin. If you've got fair skin, hair, and eyes, and normal-to-dry skin when you enter your thirties, you are likely to age much more rapidly than your darker, oilier skinned friends.

The First Signs of Aging

Because your skin's production of elastin and collagen begins to slow in your thirties, a lifetime of facial expressions will begin to show themselves in features such as frown lines, laugh lines, and crow's-feet, giving your face character. By your late thirties, gravity kicks in and you may notice, depending upon the degree of sun damage, that the skin on your neck has begun to sag.

Women, if you haven't already made or purchased a quality eye and lip makeup remover/conditioner, now is the time to do so. You need a product that will remove your makeup with minimal pulling of the delicate tissue surrounding the eye. Try my recipe for the Carrot and Calendula Complexion Conditioner on page 172. It's simple to make and has many other uses too!

Skin Care Specifics for the Thirties

- As far as I'm concerned, your saving grace for saving your face is *sunscreen!* It's as close to youth in a bottle as you can get. Use it daily!
- Wash gently — avoid overzealous scrubbing and harsh cleansers.
- Cleanse thoroughly. Rinse, rinse, rinse to remove excess cleanser and debris that can clog pores.
- Use a mild moisturizer formulated for your skin type at all times (or a sunscreen/moisturizer combination) to keep skin hydrated and prevent premature crinkling around the lips and eyes.
- Use a mild, nonabrasive exfoliant such as an alpha- or beta-hydroxy acid lotion or cream to lessen the appearance of sun damage and improve skin tone and texture.
- Throw away any makeup, lotion, cream, or aftershave that's over one year old. Products past their prime don't do your skin any favors and may be spoiled to boot.
- Throw away old makeup applicators and replace with new ones. Clean makeup and hair brushes and combs.
- Surely you're not still smoking, are you? Smoking dehydrates your skin, damages elastic tissue, and causes you to prematurely lose that tight, taut, fresh-faced look. Avoid alcohol and caffeine as well — they rob your body of nutrients and moisture.
- Relax. Destress yourself. If you're uptight, it will show up in your face as wrinkles.
- Is your whole body dry? Are you drinking plenty of fluids? Eight glasses of water and a supplement of 1 tablespoon (15 ml) of cod liver oil or flaxseed oil daily will greatly improve the condition. Slather yourself from head to toe with a quality moisturizer every day after you bathe or shower.

What's the difference between the twenties and the thirties? Just three thousand days of sun, wind, worry, and stress.

— Patricia Lone

CARROT AND CALENDULA COMPLEXION CONDITIONER

This penetrating, gentle, skin nourishing oil can also be used as a facial massage oil for all skin types except for very oily, sunburned, and couperose skin. If done on a regular basis, facial massage will increase circulation and moisture retention, resulting in smooth, glowing skin.

> 2 tablespoons (30 ml) sesame, almond, hazelnut, or jojoba oil
> 6 drops carrot seed essential oil
> 4 drops calendula essential oil

To make: Combine all ingredients in a 1-ounce (30-ml), dark glass bottle. Shake thoroughly to blend. Store in a dry, dark cabinet. For maximum potency, use within 1 year.

To remove makeup: Place a few drops onto the pad of your ring finger and apply to eyelashes or lips. You can rub the oil over your lips to dissolve any lipstick, but don't rub your eyes. Instead, close your eyes for 60 seconds and allow the oil to penetrate the lashes and break down your mascara. Ever so gently, using a moistened cotton pad and sweeping strokes from the outer corner of the eye to the inner corner, remove your makeup.

For a facial massage: One teaspoon (5 ml) of oil should be sufficient for a 5-minute facial massage before bedtime. Beginning at the base of your throat, use upward and outward strokes, progressing with sliding movements along your jawline to the base of your ears, then circular motions over your cheeks and ears and around your lips. Lightly tap around your eyes with the pads of your fingers, beginning at the outer edge and working inward. Next, beginning at the center of your forehead, use upward strokes to work your way outward with each hand, ending with circular strokes over your temples. Repeat the entire procedure up to 5 times. No need to rinse as the oil should be completely absorbed into your skin.

Yield: 1 ounce (30 ml)

THE TUMULTUOUS FORTIES

This is the decade of the midlife hormonal crisis. Your skin can be afflicted with adult acne and excess oil, then it can become as dry as the desert sands. It can be beautiful one moment, then suddenly become the bane of your existence. Women more often than men suffer from skin challenges during these years because of premenopausal symptoms. Still, men are not without their problems, as their skin does tend to show signs of dryness and reflect sun damage in the form of wrinkles around the eyes and lips. Age spots develop on their hands, arms, shoulders, and back.

As you age, your skin tone, once taut and perky, really begins to show signs of wear and tear. It loses its ability to rebound as quickly as it once did and begins to show any excesses and abuses you may have subjected it or your body to in previous years. Your muscle fibers age, or become more relaxed. Fat cells shrink. Your support network, the elastin and collagen fibers beneath the surface, begin to diminish and harden from UV exposure, nutritional deficiency, and dehydration. This loss of support occurs first in the forehead and gradually progresses downward, following gravity. Your expression lines begin to deepen and the skin on your neck and décolletage shows creases and loss of elasticity.

The First True Wrinkles

The arrival of wrinkles is a natural process resulting from a breakdown of the elastin and collagen fibers present in your skin. "Skin is a composite tissue, consisting of a fibrous matrix containing elastin and collagen. Collagen provides strength to the skin structure and elastin provides the snap or resiliency, allowing the skin to move about and assume conformational changes as required. When the elastin fibers undergo changes that cause them to lose their resiliency or snap, the skin no longer is able to return to its original state. As a result, sagging and crinkling occur in a pattern that is called wrinkles," states Peter T. Pugliese, M.D., author of *Physiology of the Skin.*

Furthermore, underlying capillaries become sclerotic (hardened), nerves die, and gravity pulls the epidermis down into the dermal layer. The superficial layer becomes thinner while the lower layers produce fewer and fewer new cells at a slower rate than when you were younger. The sebaceous glands pump less oil, also. Your skin doesn't have that youthful glow, the fresh glimmer that it once did.

The changes you began to notice in your thirties will become more pronounced in your forties. What were merely fine surface lines will now deepen and lengthen. The thin skin above and beneath your eyes may become puffy, crepey, and take on a bluish hue. Hyperpigmentation is more noticeable as age spots and uneven skin tone develop over larger areas of the body. Sun damage becomes more evident.

Men may notice that they no longer have just chest hair, but that it's crawling up and over their shoulders and sprouting on their backs as well. Don't be surprised if your significant other says you have a hair or two growing out of your ears or your nose and that your eyebrows are looking unruly

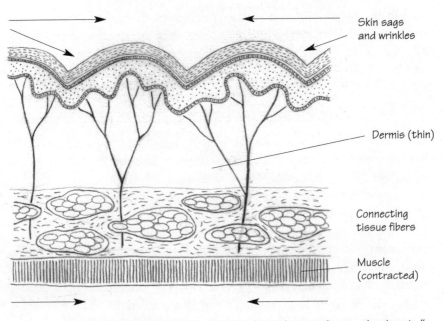

Skin sags and wrinkles

Dermis (thin)

Connecting tissue fibers

Muscle (contracted)

When elastin fibers in aging skin lose their resiliency, the dermis "sags" and folds, resulting in wrinkles.

and wiry. You can opt for this natural look or an esthetician can wax the hair on your back or your thick eyebrows if it bothers you. Nostril hair can be trimmed at home or by your barber.

Women may observe the new growth of dark hairs on their upper lip or a stray hair protruding from a mole or growing from their necks or chest. This can be disconcerting for many women, but never fear, your esthetician can wax these superfluous hairs for you or you can bleach or tweeze at home.

Skin Care Specifics for the Forties

- Sunscreen should be applied under your moisturizer and worn daily.
- The cleanser of choice should be a cleansing milk or cream so as not to strip the skin of moisture. If you have normal or oily skin, a superfatted soap bar is permissible provided you rinse thoroughly and follow with the proper moisturizer immediately.
- A good antioxidant moisturizer is a necessity unless you still have oily skin. You need a protective veil over the skin's surface to conserve the moisture you still have. Forty-plus years of exposure to the harsh elements breaks down the skin's natural defenses, so you must restore vital nutrients and moisture.
- Moisturize from head to toe, paying special attention to eyes, lips, hands, and feet. Extra care can be given to the face through soothing, hydrating facial steams, such as the recipe on page 176.
- Include an alpha- or beta-hydroxy acid treatment once or twice a week to lessen the appearance of sun damage and improve skin tone and texture.
- A good quality moisturizing mask, applied twice a week to your face, throat, and chest areas, especially during the winter months, will help to plump fine lines and wrinkles, making them less noticeable.
- Visit a dermatologist annually for a regular skin examination and check your own skin frequently. If anything seems different, have it taken care of quickly by a professional.

FACIAL STEAM

This herbal facial steam recipe was formulated by Debra St. Claire, Master Herbalist, and appears in her book, *The Herbal Medicine Cabinet.* According to Debra, "Facial steams open the pores and deep clean the tissue. They are a wonderful rejuvenator for tired skin. This formula is emollient, diaphoretic, and slightly astringent, which makes it applicable to all skin types." I found it to be quite soothing and hydrating. So to fight the ravages of day-to-day life, breathe deep of the healing vapors, and enjoy this simply glorious herbal steam!

This recipe calls for a large quantity of herbs for one facial steam, so when I made it for myself, I divided it in half and it worked just fine. This combination of herbs works well on normal skin. Recipe variations for dry and oily skin types are given following the step-by-step instructions.

1 quart (1 liter) distilled water
⅛ cup (30 ml) powdered comfrey root
⅛ cup (30 ml) powdered licorice root
⅛ cup (30 ml) peppermint leaves
⅛ cup (30 ml) chamomile flowers
⅛ cup (30 ml) calendula flowers
⅛ cup (30 ml) yarrow flowers
⅛ cup (30 ml) elderflowers
⅛ cup (30 ml) rosebuds

To make and use:
1. In a 2-quart (2-liter) saucepan, combine water, comfrey, and licorice. Allow the powders to soak for 15 minutes. Bring to a boil, then reduce heat, cover, and simmer for 10 minutes. Remove the pan from heat, add the remaining herbs, stir, cover, and let steep for 10 minutes.
2. While the herbs are steeping, do a preliminary cleansing of your face, making sure to remove all makeup. You can hold your hair away from your face with a headband.

3. Place the pan on a trivet on a table of comfortable height. Check the temperature of the steam with your hand before exposing the face. If the steam is not too hot, drape a towel over your head and shoulders and lean over the pan, letting the steam clean your face. As the mixture cools, gently blow into it to increase steam.
4. After steaming, gently pat the face dry and apply a cool astringent such as witch hazel.

To treat dry skin: Use ⅛ cup (30 ml) each of comfrey root, licorice root, marshmallow root, fennel seed, red clover flowers, and chamomile flowers.

To treat oily skin: Use ⅛ cup (30 ml) each of yarrow flowers, peppermint leaves, lemongrass, witch hazel leaves or twigs, rosebuds, lavender flowers, elderflowers, and lemon peel.

Contraindications: Do not use a facial steam if you have couperose or sunburned skin.

Yield: 1–2 treatments

FABULOUS FIFTIES

The fifties are the decade of profound physical changes in a woman's life. The most important one is menopause. From the midforties to the midfifties, a great hormonal change occurs. The production of estrogen, a female hormone that has influence on the condition of the skin, dramatically slows, causing a cessation of the menstrual cycle. As a result, women's skin becomes drier and thinner, and wrinkles become more prominent. Estrogen is also responsible for the synthesis of elastin and collagen — the substances that give skin its youthful plumpness and spring. Because of this decline in the estrogen level, women's skin will manifest a looseness, a crepey, drapey look, particularly around the eyes, jaw, nose, and throat. Men and women will notice contours change as gravity kicks in and if overweight, a double chin will likely be noticeable. The cheekbones also become more pronounced due to the shrinking of the underlying supportive fat layer. Watch for benign growths such as skin tags — thin protrusions, commonly the thickness of thin spaghetti, that extend slightly from the skin's surface — to appear on the upper body.

> *Not only does beauty fade, but it leaves a*
> *record upon the face as to what became of it.*
>
> — Elbert Hubbard

Dry Brushing

To eradicate dry skin, I recommend that both men and women adopt a simple yet invigorating morning ritual — dry brushing — for epidermal stimulation. Dry brushing revs up the circulation better than your morning cup-o-joe, guaranteed. Perfect for those of you who suffer from winter snake skin.

Dry brushing is a must for smooth, sleek, clear skin. Over the course of a day, your skin eliminates more than a pound of waste through thousands of tiny sweat glands. In fact, about one-third of all the body's impurities are excreted this way. If your pores are clogged by tight-fitting clothes, aluminum-containing antiperspirants, and mineral oil-based moisturizers, there's no way for these toxic by-products to escape. Over time, these wastes build up, causing your skin to look pale, pasty, and pimply. The dead skin cells also build up on the epidermis, resulting in a dry, flaky, lizard-like texture that forms an impenetrable barrier. Ever keep applying moisturizer over and over again to your legs and arms and still have that parched feeling, even though the bottle promises to alleviate even the most severe rough, dry skin? You have to get rid of the dead cell buildup before the moisturizer can do any good! This is where dry brushing lends a helping hand.

Contrary to what you might imagine, you can dry brush over eczema and psoriasis. Granted, you may have to lighten up on your pressure a bit, but the stimulation is superb for those thickened, scaly, rough patches.

Step 1. Dry brushing is performed on dry skin — not oiled, not damp, but dry, before you bathe or shower. Using a natural-fiber brush the size of your palm, preferably one with a handle or strap, brush your entire body, except your face (and breasts, if you're a woman), for 5 to 10 minutes. Do not brush hard. Initially, you will have to start very gently and work your way up to more vigorous brushing, but never scrub until you're red. Begin brushing your hands first, in between the fingers, then the arms, underarms, neck, chest, stomach, sides, and back. Then brush each leg, beginning with the feet. You will feel wonderfully invigorated when finished, and your skin will glow!

Step 2. Now, pour a tablespoon (15 ml) or so of sesame, almond, olive, or avocado oil into a small bowl and add a drop or two of lemongrass, German chamomile, or lavender essential oil. Massage your entire body, including your face, ears, and scalp if you're washing your hair that day. Do this for about 5 minutes. Next, jump in the shower, bathe as you usually do, and all of the dead skin you just exfoliated is washed away. Be sure to pat, not rub, your skin dry, and apply a light moisturizer after you shower.

Repeat this ritual daily. It's a good idea to wash your body brush with soap and water every week or so to keep it free of skin debris.

> *There is a case for keeping wrinkles. They are the long-service stripes earned in the hard campaign of life.*
>
> — editorial in the *London Daily Mail*

Anti-Aging Formula

▼▼▼

"This recipe," says Shatoiya de la Tour of Dry Creek Herb Farm and Learning Center, "was given to me, handed down by an old family friend from Italy. All the women in her family have lovely skin." This formula is particularly good for lightening hyperpigmentation spots, resurfacing and refining dry, flaky skin, diminishing fine lines and wrinkles (with continued use), and evening out skin tone. It works well because of the lactic acid in the yogurt and the tartaric acid in the wine. Remember, these natural acids accelerate the removal of the top layer of dead skin cells, revealing fresher, younger-looking skin.

> ½ cup (125 ml) chianti wine
> 1 cup (250 ml) fresh, thick, plain yogurt

To make: Whip wine and yogurt together in a medium-size bowl. Store any unused portion in the refrigerator for up to 2 days.

To use: It's best to do this treatment standing in the bathtub or shower stall as application can be a bit messy. Rub this mixture gently on the face as well as on rough heels, elbows, and hands. Rest for 5–15 minutes and then rinse off with water that has a splash of chianti added to it. Pat dry. Traditionally, Italian women follow this treatment with a small amount of olive oil rubbed into the skin as a moisturizer.

Yield: 1 full body treatment or several smaller spot treatments

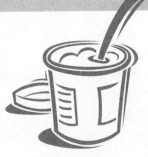

Skin Care Specifics for the Fifties

◆ The excessive sun exposure of your youth really becomes evident during this decade, so you may wish to visit your dermatologist or esthetician for glycolic acid treatments to help fade age spots and other hyperpigmented areas and to help lessen the appearance of lines and wrinkles.

◆ Sunscreen is still a daily must, especially if you are undergoing glycolic, alpha-, or beta-hydroxy acid treatments, as these products thin the epidermis and greatly increase sun sensitivity.

◆ Cleansers should be mild milks or creams unless you still have oily skin. In that case a superfatted soap bar is fine.

◆ For both men and women, a nourishing moisturizer is essential to prevent further dryness. Don't forget to apply moisturizer from head to toe.

◆ It's a good idea to keep a bottle of aromatic hydrosol handy so you can spritz your face and hair whenever you feel parched.

◆ A moisturizing mask twice a week is recommended to keep skin plump and hydrated. Avoid clay masks — they are too drying.

◆ Want to really pamper your skin? Schedule a monthly facial with your esthetician. It's an hour of luxury, but well worth it. With regular treatments you will really see a difference in the texture and clarity of your skin.

◆ Visit a dermatologist annually for regular skin examinations and check your own skin frequently. If anything seems different, have it taken care of quickly by a professional.

> *. . . for nature gives to every time and season some beauties of its own . . .*
>
> — Charles Dickens

SUPER SIXTIES

The folds, lines, and wrinkles evident in your fifties are now even more noticeable, due to loss of muscle tone and the continued shrinkage of the subcutaneous layer. Sagging, drooping tissue above your eyes may make them appear smaller and not as bright and expressive as they once were.

Moisture retention is key as you get older. As the body ages, it loses moisture overall. Unless moisture is replenished internally through diet and externally through the application of good moisturizers, existing lines and wrinkles will deepen at a rapid pace. My advice is to make sure you always consume plenty of water each day, eat a diet that's high in water content (lots of fresh fruits and vegetables), eliminate all diuretics (coffee, cola drinks, black tea), add a tablespoon (15 ml) of flaxseed oil or cod liver oil and perhaps a 500 mg capsule of evening primrose or borage oil to your diet, dry brush, and moisturize every day.

Caring for Your Scalp

The skin on your head, your scalp, is often ignored, but it needs just as much care as the rest of your body in order to function properly and look its best. With the sweat glands shrinking and the sebaceous glands pumping less lubricating oil, many of you in your sixties will suffer from thinning, dry hair and dry scalp, especially if you have colored your hair for some time or have been using harsh shampoos and styling products.

Women in this age group often experience thinning hair, especially at the crown, due to hormonal influences related to menopause. Men may be genetically predisposed to male-pattern baldness or have stress-related hair loss. Natural thinning can also occur with age, as the hair follicles begin to shrink and produce thinner, finer hairs with a shorter lifespan.

Melanie Von Zabuesnig, an aromatherapist specializing in hair care and issues relating to hair loss, is the owner of VZ Botanicals (see resources). At thirty-two she had a rare scalp disorder, alopecia areata, that caused all her hair, even

Scalp Conditioner and Stimulator

The oils in this formula can help add shine and moisture to dry hair and stimulate hair growth. The lemon and grapefruit essential oils create an uplifting effect on the user while stimulating growth, regulating sebum production, and encouraging cell regeneration. The uplifting effect is an added benefit that makes the formula more tempting to use!

This formula will help to get the scalp in the best possible condition by cleansing the scalp and nourishing the hair roots. It usually takes a minimum of 3 months to see noticeable new growth. Many people notice a drastic improvement in texture and appearance much sooner, even after the first use!

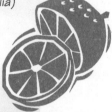

- 2 teaspoons (10 ml) lavender (*Lavandula angustifolia*) essential oil
- 1 teaspoon (5 ml) geranium essential oil
- 1 teaspoon (5 ml) ylang-ylang essential oil (for a sweet fragrance)
- 1 teaspoon (5 ml) lemon essential oil
- 1 teaspoon (5 ml) grapefruit essential oil
- 2 teaspoons (10 ml) yarrow essential oil (optional, for more serious thinning problems)
- 3 tablespoons (45 ml) pure, unrefined jojoba oil

To make: Mix all ingredients together in a 4-ounce (120-ml) dark glass bottle. Shake well. Store in a dry, dark cabinet for up to 1 year.

To use: Massage 1 teaspoon (5 ml) into scalp with your fingertips for 3 minutes. Leave on for 1 hour or longer to allow oils to penetrate (can be left on overnight). Wash out with a natural shampoo. Use this treatment 2–3 times per week.

Yield: Approximately 15 treatments

her eyelashes, to fall out. Her aromatherapy formulas brought it back, thick and healthy. The Scalp Conditioner and Stimulator on page 183 is one of her recipes that she has kindly let me share with you.

Skin Care Specifics for the Sixties

- Basically you'll want to keep doing what you did in your fifties (see page 181). However, at this age skin cancer becomes more prevalent, so you must keep a vigilant eye on any skin growths or unusual skin discolorations that crop up.
- If diagnosed with skin cancer, please heed your physician's advice and stay out of the sun or at least be well protected from head to toe.
- A little extra weight — not a lot, mind you — is beneficial as far as appearances go. A bit of fat on your body has a way of smoothing out those encroaching wrinkles. If thin or sickly at this age, skin tends to hang, causing you to look older than you should.
- Mature skin can benefit from a nonabrasive exfoliating mask to prevent dead skin cell buildup, such as a green papaya enzyme mask (available from September's Sun Herbal Soap & Skin Care Company) or the Anti-Aging Formula (page 180).
- Pay extra attention to your diet. Make sure you consume plenty of antioxidants, fats, proteins, complex carbohydrates, and fiber.
- Don't forget to exercise for health and stress relief. The more oxygen available to your system, the better your skin looks and feels.

If man is moderate and contented, then even age is no burden; if he is not, then even youth is full of cares.

— Plato

STILL RADIANT IN YOUR
SEVENTIES AND BEYOND

From approximately the midsixties onward, the bones of the skull begin to shrink, yet the skin still grows; this leads to sagging. The underlying supportive elastin and collagen fibers have gone into retirement, so the entire face and body appear to simply be hanging around, droopy and wrinkly. If you're overweight or muscular, there is a bit of cushioning for your skin to grab on to. The fullness of your cheeks and chin is no longer there because the fat padding is being absorbed and the bones becoming more prominent. Your epidermis, now only a thin veneer of what it once was, is no longer working at its youthful capacity.

However, not everyone at this age looks the worse for wear. Many people actually get better looking with age, and depending on how well you cared for yourself in the past decades, you may be chronologically seventy-plus years of age, but your biological age may be closer to fifty! Remember, photoaging or environmental aging, poor nutrition, excessive stress, and lack of exercise can add years to your appearance.

At this age, your skin has experienced a little bit of everything under the sun, and then some. Sure, you still want to protect it from further environmental damage, but your main concern is hydrating, nurturing, and preventing dryness. Many people, women in particular, find that they bruise much more easily now than they ever have. Unfortunately, as the years pass, the epidermal layer and fat padding thins, becoming less effective at cushioning everyday assaults. The capillaries are much closer to the surface, too, so it doesn't take much to cause subcutaneous hemorrhaging. Healing takes place at a slower pace as well.

Aging Gracefully

According to the American Academy of Dermatology, "The prevalence of skin disease increases throughout our lives. Most people past age seventy have at least one skin problem, many develop three or four. But with proper management, our skin can remain healthy so we can look as good as we feel."

The thinning of the epidermis just reinforces the constant battle with dry skin. Try the dry brushing technique mentioned on page 178. It greatly benefits all skin types.

For your daily massage or bath, try one of these penetrating and nourishing bath and body oils to help combat dry skin:

- Avocado
- Hazelnut
- Jojoba
- Almond
- Sesame
- Coconut

Use 1 tablespoon (15 ml) in the bath or 1 to 2 tablespoons (15–30 ml) as a massage oil.

Sunflower Friction

One of my favorite body and facial scrubs to use during the winter months is a superfatted mixture of raw sunflower kernels and heavy cream. It's high in emollients and is an excellent makeup remover (keep away from eye area). Try this recipe and see if your skin doesn't feel like velvet!

1 tablespoon (15 ml) finely ground raw sunflower kernels
1 tablespoon (15 ml) heavy cream

To make: In a small bowl, combine ingredients until a spreadable paste forms.

To use: Apply scrub to face, neck, and chest, gently massaging in circular motions for about 2 minutes. Rinse. I like to do this in the shower or while leaning over the bathtub or sink as it can be a bit messy. It never seems to clog my drain, though. If you want to scrub your whole body, triple or quadruple the recipe according to your size. This recipe can be used daily if you wish, even on the most sensitive of skins.

Yield: 1 treatment

PURE CREAM CLEANSER

This simple cleanser is perfect for all skin types, except oily. It's wonderfully emollient, leaves skin soft and hydrated, and even removes eye and lip makeup. Tastes good, too! All the benefits of real cream without making you fat.

1 tablespoon (15 ml) heavy cream
1 drop carrot seed or rose essential oil
   (Use the rose oil if you're feeling indulgent!)

To make: Mix ingredients thoroughly in a small bowl.
To use: Apply cream blend with a flannel cloth or soft washcloth in gentle circular motions over entire face, neck, and chest. Rinse. Pat dry. Follow with your favorite toner and moisturizer if you desire.
Yield: 1 treatment

Skin Care Specifics for the Seventies and Beyond

◆ Follow the skin care recommendations for the sixties listed on page 184.
◆ Accept yourself for the beauty or character you've become. Realize that your skin cells don't regenerate themselves as rapidly as they once did and that no matter what topical treatments you use, whether natural, chemical, or surgical, your skin will continue to show signs of advanced aging. Science has not figured out a way to make us grow young again — at least not yet! Granted, a dermatologist can offer various treatments that can improve the appearance and condition of your skin remarkably, but at a price. Your esthetician can be of assistance as well, though, to a lesser degree.

Suggested Reading

Airola, Paavo, N.D. *How To Get Well*. Phoenix, AZ: Health Plus Publishers, 1974.

Balin, Arthur K., M.D., Ph.D., and Loretta Pratt Balin, M.D. *The Life of the Skin: What It Hides, What It Reveals, and How It Communicates*. New York: Bantam Books, 1997.

Bremness, Lesley. *Herbs*. New York: Dorling Kindersley Publishing, 1994.

Castleman, Michael. *The Healing Herbs: The Ultimate Guide to the Curative Power of Nature's Medicine*. Emmaus, PA: Rodale Press, 1991.

Chase, Deborah. *Fruit Acids for Fabulous Skin*. New York: St. Martin's Press, 1996.

Garrison, Robert H., Jr., M.A., R.Ph., and Elizabeth Somer, M.A., R.D. *The Nutrition Desk Reference*. New Canaan, CT: Keats Publishing, 1985.

Gerson, Joel. *Standard Textbook for Professional Estheticians: techniques for skin care and makeup specialists*. 5th edition. New York, NY: MILADY Publishing Corporation, 1986.

Irons, Diane. *The World's Best-Kept Beauty Secrets*. Naperville, IL: Sourcebooks, 1997.

Jonas, Wayne, and Jennifer Jacobs. *Healing with Homeopathy: The Doctor's Guide*. New York: Warner Books, 1998.

Keville, Kathi. *Herbs for Health and Healing: A Drug-Free Guide to Prevention and Cure*. Emmaus, PA: Rodale Press, 1996.

Kirschmann, John D., and Lavon J. Dunne. *Nutrition Almanac*. 2nd ed. New York: McGraw-Hill Book Company, 1984.

Lavabre, Marcel. *Aromatherapy Workbook*. Rochester, VT: Healing Arts Press, 1990.

Lust, John B., N.D., D.B.M. *The Herb Book*. New York: Bantam Books, 1974.

Parentini, Lynn J. *The Joy of Healthy Skin: A Lifetime Guide to Beautiful Problem-Free Skin*. Englewood Cliffs, NJ: Prentice Hall, 1996.

Pugliese, Peter T., M.D. *Physiology of the Skin*. Carol Stream, IL: Allured Publishing Corporation, 1996.

Raichur, Pratima. *Absolute Beauty: Radiant Skin and Inner Harmony through the Ancient Secrets of Ayurveda*. New York: HarperCollins, 1997.

St. Claire, Debra, M.H. *The Herbal Medicine Cabinet*. Berkeley, CA: Celestial Arts, 1998.

Schnaubelt, Kurt. *Aromatherapy Course*. 2nd ed. San Rafael, CA: Pacific Institute of Aromatherapy.

Sheats, Cliff. *Lean Bodies: The Revolutionary New Approach to Losing Bodyfat by Increasing Calories*. Fort Worth, TX: The Summit Group, 1992.

Steen, Edwin B., and Ashley Montagu. *Anatomy and Physiology*, Volume 1. 2nd ed. New York: Harper & Row, 1984.

Stone, Robert, and Webster Stone. *Zit Wars: the battle for great skin*. New York: Arbor House Publishing, 1986.

Tortora, Gerard J., and Nicholas P. Anagnostakos. *Principles of Anatomy and Physiology*. 4th ed. New York: Harper & Row, 1984.

Weiss, Gaea, and Shandor Weiss. *Growing & Using the Healing Herbs*. Emmaus, PA: Rodale Press, 1985.

Worwood, Valerie Ann. *The Complete Book of Essential Oils & Aromatherapy*. San Rafael, CA: New World Library, 1991.

RESOURCES

Herbs and Natural Products

The American Botanical Pharmacy
P.O. Box 3027
Santa Monica, CA 90408
Info: (310) 453-1987
Orders: (888) 437-2362
Organically grown and wild-harvested herbal preparations. Highly recommended! Free catalog.

Aura Cacia
P.O. Box 299
Norway, IA 52318
(800) 437-3301
Source for quality essential oils and related items. Free catalog.

Champlain Valley Apiaries
Box 127
Middlebury, VT 05753-0127
(800) 841-7334
Fax: (802) 388-1653
Owned by W.A. Mraz. Excellent source for reasonably priced raw honey, maple syrup, and beeswax. Free brochure.

Dry Creek Herb Farm and Learning Center
13935 Dry Creek Road
Auburn, CA 95602
(530) 878-2441
Fax: (530) 878-6772
High-quality organically grown herbs. Free catalog.

Fredericksburg Herb Farm
P.O. Drawer 927
Fredericksburg, TX 78624-0927
(800) 259-HERB
Fax: (830) 997-5069
E-mail: herbfarm@ktc.com
Website:
www.fredericksburgherbfarm.com
This herb farm, tea room, and day spa is must see! An oasis under the hot Texas sun! Their free catalog carries many herbal bath and body products as well as delicious herbal tea blends.

The Great Cape Cod Herb, Spice & Tea Co.
2628 Main Street
P.O. Box 1206
Brewster, MA 02631
(508) 896-5900
(800) 427-7144
Fax: (508) 896-1972
E-mail: ginkgo@greatcape.com
Web site: www.greatcape.com
This is Stephan Brown's company. Complete old-fashioned herbal apothecary. Free catalog.

Janca's Jojoba Oil and Seed Company
456 E. Juanita #7
Mesa, Arizona 85204
(602) 497-9494
Fax: (602) 497-1312
Fine-quality jojoba oil, base oils, essential oils, cosmetic butters, herbs, waxes, cosmetic chemicals and cosmetics, soap and candle making supplies, bottles, jars, bags, etc. Free catalog.

Jean's Greens Herbal Tea Works!!
119 Sulphur Spring Road
Norway, NY 13416
(315) 845-6500
(888) 845-TEAS
Fax: (315) 845-6501
E-mail: jean@jeansgreens.com
Web site: www.jeansgreens.com
Jean Argus, the owner, is a wonderful woman. Her shop carries just about everything you'll need for the remedies in this book. Reasonable prices, friendly service. Free catalog.

Liberty Natural Products
8120 SE Stark Street
Portland, OR 97215-2346
(800) 289-8427
Offers a variety of herbal extracts, essential oils, and natural products. Free catalog.

LorAnn Oils
4518 Aurelius Road
P.O. Box 22009
Lansing, MI 48909-2009
(888) 456-7266
Fax: (517) 882-0507
Web site: www.lorannoils.com
Homemade candy and soap supplies, essential oils, base oils, wax, fragrance oils, and other natural products. Free catalog.

Morningstar Publications
44 Rim Road
Boulder, CO 80302
(303) 444-6072
Fax: (303) 473-9997
Operated by Debra St. Claire, Master Herbalist. Offers a videotape set, Herbal Preparations & Natural Therapies: Creating and Using a Home Herbal Medicine Chest. *Step-by-step instructions show how to make many useful herbal formulations. Highly recommended!*

Mountain Rose Herbs
20818 High Street
North San Juan, CA 95960
(800) 879-3337
Fax: (530) 292-9138
Web site: www.botanical.com/mtrose
Herbs, herb seeds, base oils, essential oils, bottles, jars, hair and skin care products, tinctures, salves, and teas. Free catalog.

Original Swiss Aromatics
P.O. Box 6842
San Rafael, CA 94903
(415) 459-3998
Fax: (415) 479-0614
Superior-quality "genuine & authentic" (g&a) and vintage essential oils. They specialize in providing absolutely genuine essential oils from farmers and distillers. Their oils are guaranteed pure and suitable for aromatherapy work or other healing modalities. Free catalog.

Pacific Institute of Aromatherapy
P.O. Box 6723
San Rafael, CA 94903
(415) 479-9121
Fax: (415) 479-0119
Superior-quality essential oils and indepth aromatherapy certification correspondence course and seminars. Free catalog.

September's Sun Herbal Soap and Skin Care Company
Stephanie Tourles, Owner
P.O. Box 772
West Hyannisport, MA 02672
(508) 862-9955
Fax: (508) 778-9262
Handmade herbal/grain-based soaps and goat milk soaps, herbal body products, Super Blue Green™ Algae, and personally signed herb books. Send SASE for free product brochure.

Seventh Generation
Gaiam, Inc.
360 Interlocken Boulevard, Suite 300
Broomfield, CO 80021
(800) 456-1177
Fax: (800) 456-1139
Offers naturally-based products for cleansing your home and body, and fragrance-free and dye-free cotton bed and bath goods. Many other unique items. Good resource for those with allergies. Free catalog.

Simplers Botanical Co.
P.O. Box 2534
Sebastopol, CA 95473
(800) 652-7646
Fax: (707) 887-7570
Pharmaceutical-grade essential oils, tinctures, glycerites, aromatic hydrosols, herbal skin care products, and books. Excellent essential oils for the aromatherapist or skin care professional. Free catalog.

Sunburst Bottle Co.
5710 Auburn Blvd. #7
Sacramento, CA 95841
(916) 348-5576
Fax: (916) 348-3803
Web site: www.sunburstbottle.com
Offers every type of bottle or jar you'll ever need. Reasonably priced, no minimums. Free catalog.

VZ Botanicals
24046 Crowned Partridge Lane
Murrietta, CA 92562
(909) 677-1318
Fax: (909) 677-9558
E-mail: vz@earthlink.net
A mail-order business, owned by Melanie Von Zabuesnig, operated through the internet. Specializes in essential oil blends for alopecia patients.

Helpful Organizations

American Academy of Dermatology
P.O. Box 4014
Schaumburg, IL 60168-4014
(888) 462-DERM
Fax: (847) 330-8907
Web site: www.aad.org
Call for physician referrals and free informative skin care brochures.

American Cancer Society
1599 Clifton Road, N.E.
Atlanta, GA 30329
(800) ACS-2345
Web site: www.cancer.org
Call for skin care and skin cancer brochures.

American Herb Association
P.O. Box 1673
Nevada City, CA 95959
(530) 265-9552
Excellent newsletter. Send for free brochure.

Herb Research Foundation
1007 Pearl Street, Suite 200
Boulder, CO 80302
Orders only: (800) 307-6267
Other inquiries: (303) 449-2265
Fax: (303) 449-7849
E-mail: info@herbs.org
Web site: www.herbs.org
A nonprofit research and education center dedicated to providing up-to-date, unbiased information on the health benefits and safety of medicinal plants. Membership includes a magazine subscription, quarterly newsletter, and discounts on all HRF information services. Send for free brochure.

National Eczema Association for Science and Education
1221 S.W. Yamhill, Suite 303
Portland, OR 97205
(800) 818-7546
(503) 228-4430
Fax: (503) 273-8778
Newsletter, educational materials, and support group information.

National Psoriasis Foundation
6600 S.W. 92nd Avenue, Suite 300
Portland, OR 97223-7195
(800) 723-9166
Fax: (503) 245-0626
E-mail: getinfo@npfusa.org
Web site: http://www.psoriasis.org
Call for informational brochures.

National Rosacea Society
800 South Northwest Highway, Suite 200-R
Barrington, IL 60010
Fax: (847) 382-5567
A nonprofit organization publishing the "Rosacea Review" newsletter. Send for free subscription.

Northeast Herbal Association
P.O. Box 10
Newport, NY 13416
E-mail: neha@jeansgreens.com
A wonderful herbal networking organization for the exchange of topics of importance to the herbal community. Membership includes a super tri-annual newsletter. Send for information.

The Science and Art of Herbology
Sage Mountain
P.O. Box 420
East Barre, VT 05649
(802) 479-9825
Offers a superior herbal correspondence course and residential programs, taught by Rosemary Gladstar. Highly recommended! Send a large SASE for information.

The Skin Cancer Foundation
P.O. Box 561
New York, NY 10156
(800) 754-6490
(212) 725-5176
Fax: (212) 725-5751
E-mail: info@skincancer.org
Call for informative skin cancer brochures.

Therapeutic Herbalism
2068 Ludwig Avenue
Santa Rosa, CA 95407
Another highly recommended herbal correspondence course. Send a large SASE for course information.

United Plant Savers
P.O. Box 420
East Barre, VT 05649
A nonprofit organization that compiles information on threatened or endangered medicinal plants, provides resources for replanting and restoration projects, secures land trusts for the preservation of plant diversity, and raises public awareness about the overharvesting of precious medicinal herbs. Send a large SASE for an informational brochure.

INDEX

Entries in **boldface** indicate recipes;
page references in *italics* indicate illustrations.

S

Sage *(Salvia officinalis)*, 24, 62

Salves, 152

   Comfrey/Calendula Healing Salve, 140–141, 144–145, 152

Scalp, care for, 182–184

Scalp Conditioner and Stimulator, 183

Scars, 150–153

Scrapes, 106–108

Sea salt, 65

   Ocean Potion bath, 117

Seasonal variations

   skin protection for, 112

   various skin types, 23, 25–29

Sebaceous glands, 23, 24, 85, 174

Sebum, 23, 26, 75–77, 85

   decrease with aging, 170, 174

   maintenance, 82

   normalizing production of, 79

   Sebum Balancing Formula, 82

Seeds, 17, 56–57

Sensitive skin, 28–29

Sesame oil, 44

Seventies and beyond, 185–187

Shaving irritations, 154–158, *154*

Silicon, 9, 149

Sixties, skin care for, 182–184

Skin

   basics of care, 21–31, 40

   function, 5

   structure, 1–4, *3*

   types of, 23–30

Skin Ailment Assailment Tea, 140–143

Skin cancer, 89–96, 184

   identifying, 92–93, *92–93*

   self-examination, 94–95

Skin examinations

   annual check-ups, 175, 181

   cancer self-examination, 94–95

   professional facial, 35, 37

Skin-Sational herb tea, 12

Skin-So-Smoothie, 13

Skin tags, 178

Skin Tea, 149

Sleep, 79, 120, 121

Smoking, 30, 168, 171

Soap

   for poison ivy, oak, sumac, 136

   as skin cleanser, 23, 25, 26, 27, 28, 29

Soothing Eye Compress, 122

Soothing Licorice Tea, 118

Soybean oil, 44

Spices, 57–62

Spicy Aftershave, 157

Spike lavender *(Lavandula spica)* essential oil, 26, 29, 51

St.-John's-wort, 144, 152

Steam treatment. *See* Facial steams

Strawberry, 55

Stress, 40, 85, 86, 129, 184

   acne and, 77, 78

   aging, effect on, 168, 171

   eczema and, 116

   herpes, role in, 125–126

   rosacea, cause of, 147

   visual, 120

Subcutaneous tissue, 3, 4

Sulfur, 9

Sunburn, 159–163

   Aloe After-Sun Relief Spray, 162

   Sunburn Relief For Children, 163

Sunflower, 56–57

   Sunflower Friction, 186

Sunlight, 20, 31, 131, 184. *See also* Skin cancer

   photoaging from, 165–166

   psoriasis treatment, 139

Sunscreen, 20, 22, 31, 40, 89, 94, 121, 160–161, 168, 171, 175, 181

Supplements, 11–20

   acne treatment, 78

   Apricot Chews, 16

   couperose complexion treatment, 106

   eczema treatment, 116

   herpes treatment, 126–127

   hives treatment, 130

   Honey Pecan Cookies, 15

   poison ivy, oak, sumac prevention, 136

   rosacea treatment, 149, 150

   Skin-Sational Herb Tea, 12

   Skin-So-Smoothie, 13

   Sweet 'N' Nutty Snack Mix, 17

Sweet 'N' Nutty Snack Mix, 17